Jim Horne is Professor of Psychophysiology and Director of the Sleep Research Centre at Loughborough University, UK. He is a fellow of the Institute of Biology and the British Psychological Society, and is Editor-in-Chief of the *Journal of Sleep Research*. He is frequently called upon to discuss topics related to sleep on radio and television, and writes regularly for the broadsheets and for scientific magazines. His previous books include *Why We Sleep* (1988, OUP).

To Rosie, George and Helen

Sleepfaring

A journey through the science of sleep

JIM HORNE

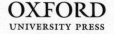

OXFORD
UNIVERSITY PRESS

OXFORD
UNIVERSITY PRESS

Great Clarendon Street, Oxford OX2 6DP

Oxford University Press is a department of the University of Oxford.
It furthers the University's objective of excellence in research, scholarship,
and education by publishing worldwide in

Oxford New York

Auckland Cape Town Dar es Salaam Hong Kong Karachi
Kuala Lumpur Madrid Melbourne Mexico City Nairobi
New Delhi Shanghai Taipei Toronto

With offices in

Argentina Austria Brazil Chile Czech Republic France Greece
Guatemala Hungary Italy Japan Poland Portugal Singapore
South Korea Switzerland Thailand Turkey Ukraine Vietnam

Oxford is a registered trade mark of Oxford University Press
in the UK and in certain other countries

Published in the United States
by Oxford University Press Inc., New York

First published 2006
First published as an Oxford University Paperback 2007

British Library Cataloguing in Publication Data

Data available

Library of Congress Cataloging in Publication Data

Data available

Typeset by RefineCatch Limited, Bungay, Suffolk
Printed in Great Britain by
Clays Ltd, St Ives plc
ISBN 978–0–19–922837–9

1 3 5 7 9 10 8 6 4 2

Contents

Preface

Many people view sleep as a rather mysterious way of eliminating sleepiness. Not so much the elixir of life perhaps, but maybe it removes a few wrinkles and those 'bags under the eyes'. If only there was a pill to abolish both sleep and sleepiness, then we could add half as much again to our waking lives. No more time wasting in preparing for bed each night, save money on a smaller house without bedrooms, and all that free time for entertainment, socialising, and surfing the internet. No need to lose sleep over insomnia, no more sleep-related road crashes, freedom to fly at night without noise restrictions, and all that extra time with our ever-active kids who will not be sleeping either. Ah, there's a thought—maybe not such a sweet dream after all, but more of a nightmare, as a sleepless world would be a relentless one, everyone on the go, working round the clock, and with little time to chill out by oneself.

Sleep is not like the bedside light—a simple click and off to oblivion. It is such an intricate process, involving so many parts and substances within the brain, that to do away with it would require a hitherto incomprehensible potpourri of drugs, which is why sleep is so intriguing. Besides, it dominates our lives and is far from being a soporific subject, and from what little we still know it is well beyond the fantasy of dreams.

'What? There's no such word' is the usual response to the title of this book—Sleepfaring. It rolls off the tongue, though, and sticks in the mind when I explain that 'fare' is from the old English '*fær*' (travel or journey), and that mine is a journey through the science and practice of sleep, or lack of it. What is more, 'fare' relates to health ('how fare ye?'), and sleep is intimately tied up with health, well-being, and, especially, one's welfare. Enough on this point, except to say that as 'fare' is also linked to being entertained and fed, 'sleepfaring' has its lighter as well as its serious moments.

Even the simplest of all living organisms have regular, daily rest periods, overseen by an internal 'body clock'. But when does rest become sleep? Bees, scorpions, and squid certainly sleep because, for them, it brings unconsciousness. What of plants at night, when photosynthesis ceases—are they unconscious? For humans and fellow mammals, the role of sleep will differ, depending on body size and complexity of the brain—from being an energy-conserving immobiliser for the mouse, to the sole provider of rest for the higher centres of the human brain. This is the theme of Chapter 1—the purpose of sleep. But who is 'half asleep', and what about the ungainly giraffe and the one-eyed duck? Chapter 2 homes in on the human brain, which only comprises two to three per cent of our body weight, but it is relatively huge—not so much in size, perhaps, but in its demands. When awake it consumes a fifth of both the oxygen that we breathe and the calories that we eat. Unlike all other organs, able to rest when we relax in front of the TV, the 'human' parts of our brain cannot rest like this, but only during sleep. The chapter ends with a twist to 'sleeping like a baby'. Chapter 3 likens sleep to a car journey and the substances within the sleeping brain to a cocktail, recommends eating as a bed partner for sleep, and finally takes its leave of you in a coffee house.

All too easily forgotten are the fascinating early pioneering experiments into sleep, revived in Chapter 4. Although maybe rather crude by today's standards, they still have much to contribute. In some respects all we have done since then is to repeat them, with similar outcomes. Chapter 5 describes how sleep loss turns us into automatons working on 'autopilot', but the occasionally odd behaviour is not a sign of madness. Moreover, sleep loss can even be therapeutic.

'Do we grow in our sleep?' is the topic of Chapter 6, although it is mostly a matter of shrinking during wakefulness. Findings with beauty sleep, disappearing wrinkles, perspiration, and 'night starvation' come under the microscope, as do the growth of body cells and what happens to our immune system—all of which can all too easily be misinterpreted.

Measurement of sleepiness, the subject of Chapter 7, ranges from self-insight, and looking at the eyes, to the monitoring of 'lapses' and brain waves, but not to counting yawns, though. None of this is straightforward, because sleepiness, like hunger, is influenced by 'mind over matter' and boredom. Chapter 8 reveals how our thought processes are affected by sleepiness, with sleepy doctors and executives having difficulty in diagnosing and decision-making—can they really cope with emergencies? Sleep loss mimics the ageing brain—which is not to say that older people are particularly sleepy, because the antidote for the ageing mind is to keep it busy.

Literally, the greatest impact of sleepiness is from falling asleep at the wheel, and the theme for Chapter 9. The body clock plays a crucial role, as do even small amounts of alcohol when combined with sleepiness. Sleepy drivers know that they are sleepy—so why do they carry on driving, and are they responsible for what may happen? Better news comes with practical advice for drivers on how to combat this sleepiness.

It is time for the body clock in Chapters 10 and 11. Called the 'circadian rhythm', its daily highs and lows are reflected in both body and behaviour, although differing between 'larks' and 'owls'. Rate yourself on the lark–owl questionnaire! There is a bath to be taken with the explanation of how wakefulness and this clock affect the length and timing of sleep. Melatonin, the hormone of the night, is not so dark and mysterious in the way that it alters the body clock. Judicious lighting helps with shift work and jetlag, and there is advice on coping with both. Is shift work harmful? As for moonlighting, it is not what you think.

At last, to sleep, in Chapters 12 and 13. When do young and old, and men and women, go to bed and get up, and for how long do they sleep? About five times an hour we move during sleep, but when does this become 'tossing and turning'? 'Brain waves' are the window on the sleeping brain, but then there are those eponymous 'rapid eye movements' of REM or 'dreaming' sleep. Both provide the basis for the 'hypnogram', showing how light, deep, and REM sleep alternate over the night. What is 'brain strain', and why is a warm bath as good as a physical work-out in improving sleep? How come sight seeing is so exhausting, and what about those aching feet?

The enigma of REM sleep comes not from the accompanying dreams, but from whether it is sleep at all. Is it a type of wakefulness or 'non-wakefulness', similar to a computer in 'screen-saver' mode? So goes the debate in Chapters 14 and 15. The abundance of REM sleep in early life points to its real role—in stimulating the developing brain. Why are we paralysed and emotionless during REM sleep? Nevertheless, it is fairly dispensable and mental health might be better without it.

Dreams are the 'cinema of the mind'—merely best-forgotten B movies, argues Chapter 16. There are lots of fascinating facts and plenty of fiction, here, with the fantasising being in dream interpretation rather than with the dreamer. What about 'lucid dreams'—are these confused with other forms of imagery appearing on the boundaries between sleep and wakefulness?

'How much sleep do we need?' is the hot topic for Chapters 17 and 18. Are long and short sleepers really healthy? What is the 'more or less' of sleep, and can we sleep to excess? Is our 'sleep debt' any worse today than yesteryear, and do laboratory tests paint the real picture? 'Tiredness' and 'sleepiness' are not synonymous, and maybe we should be taking more exercise instead of extra sleep.

Insomnia is the enigma for Chapters 19 and 20. What are its causes, how sleepless are people with insomnia, how does it change with age, do women suffer more than men, and what about elderly people—is their early morning awakening really insomnia? Not sleepy in the day? Then is your insomnia really a disorder of sleep or, rather, one of wakefulness? Plenty of advice, here, but what about the bed—that is a 'great' story.

There is nothing amusing about 'heroic snoring', more imposingly called 'obstructive sleep apnoea'—a gross disturbance of sleep causing excessive daytime sleepiness and the focus of Chapter 21. Obesity is a common culprit, but there is a quicker remedy than slimming. Such snoring contrasts with the silent but equally debilitating 'restless' or 'jerky' legs—so easily overlooked, but not here.

Last, but not least, children's sleep is scrutinised in Chapter 22. What is normal sleep? Getting off to sleep, failure to 'self-sooth', and interrupted sleep present many predicaments, all too often and unwittingly of the parents' own making, although more easily overcome than imagined. Sleepwalking, sleep terrors, nightmares, head banging, bedwetting, sleep talking, tooth grinding, and snoring are more of the topics to be found. Today's bedroom is likely to be festooned with electronic goodies, serving only to postpone bedtime and shorten sleep. Sleepy children may not seem sleepy, but inattentive, bad tempered, and hyperactive—sometimes mistaken for mild attention deficit disorder.

These are only some of the landmarks to be encountered in your forthcoming journey through sleep. The route I shall be taking is not typical, and many of the views will be different, but the scenery is marvellous, nevertheless. So, come aboard, the course is set and the tide is turning—bon voyage!

Jim Horne

List of figures and tables

Petunias, one-eyed ducks, and roly-poly mice

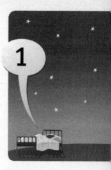

Do plants sleep?

All living organisms, including bacteria and plants, have a regular, daily period of rest and inactivity, but whether this can be seen as sleep is another matter. Plants cease their photosynthesis at night, not simply because of the dark but because, like all other living organisms, they have their own daily internal 'biological clock', called a circadian rhythm (from the Latin *circa* about, *diem* day). *Sanservia*, the 'sensitive plant', closes its leaves when touched and also closes them at night. Nevertheless, if it is kept in the dark continuously, the leaves will persist in opening during normal daylight hours. But to say that plants sleep is not only a 'leap in the dark' but remains a leap of faith if one thinks about whether they can be woken up or whether they become 'unconscious', which are the keys to real sleep. The idea of waking a petunia, a hedge, or even a cactus for that matter, is of course bizarre. Whereas we can 'sleep like a log', ironically, a tree probably cannot do so.

Bacteria move about and multiply in a daily manner governed by their biological clocks, and show distinct, regular periods of inactivity. Even amoebae, the simplest of all animals, with their single body cell that moves by protruding and withdrawing parts of its surface ('pseudopodia'), regularly turns into an inactive blob, often at night, and can stay like this for hours, even if gently poked. Is it asleep or is it simply having a rest and refusing to budge?

For more advanced animals, the unconsciousness of sleep makes them less responsive, although even the deepest sleeper can be stirred into action by danger, which makes sleep different from anaesthesia or from simply being knocked out. Sleep, rather than rest, and when

1

the term 'unconsciousness' can be used, is certainly to be found in insects. For example, at night the bee sleeps for about 6–8 hours, when it will often roll over on its side, have 'droopy' antennae, and be fairly unresponsive to other bees bumping into it. Although most insects have very good eyes, there are no eyelids, and so we cannot tell from their eyes whether they are asleep. However, as antennae are just as important as eyes, and probably more so, droopy antennae certainly indicate that the animal is not in contact with reality and is not just resting. Bees[1] as well as flies[2] can easily be sleep deprived by keeping them in continuously moving jars, so that the insects have to fly about all the time. When the jar stops moving they settle down and are even less responsive than normal to further, gentle shaking of the jar. It is as if their sleep has become deeper in compensation for its loss.

Professor Irene Tobler, from Zurich University, has studied the sleep of more animals than anyone else, most notably in scorpions.[3] When sleeping they can (gently!) be picked up without their stirring—the skill, she confidently tells me, is to know when they are really asleep rather than just sitting still, ready to attack!

The octopus and cuttle-fish certainly sleep, and not only do they become immobile and unresponsive but also their skins go crinkly and change into characteristic and attractive colour patterns, almost as if saying 'I'm asleep'. The patterns may be cute and attractive to us but are a warning to predators. These animals do not have eyelids either, although their pupils become particularly narrow during sleep and somehow can still spot danger. This is certainly sleep because, like many other animals, if they are kept awake they will compensate by sleeping more later on.

Readers with goldfish or tropical fish may notice that at night they go to the same spot in the aquarium and stay there fairly motionless, often for several hours. Even dropping food into the tank will usually produce little response. In their wild state fish will retire to a favourite, but safe, area among weeds or rocks. More unusual is the parrot fish, which inhabits more exposed areas of sea and has to create its own protection when sleeping. It does this by secreting around its body a slimy envelope, which is distasteful to predators. In the morning it packs its bags, so to speak, by eating the envelope. Sleeping fish usually remain still but carry on breathing by 'gulping' water and forcing it through their gills. On the other hand, most sleeping sharks usually cannot stay motionless like this, and have to keep moving, slowly and aimlessly, to push rather than gulp water through their gills.

Migrating birds and albatrosses at sea fly for days at a time. Whether they can somehow 'sleep on the wing', or just deprive themselves of sleep, is a matter that remains to be discovered, although the answer probably favours 'sleep deprivation'—as laboratory studies[4] show that they can go for long periods without sleep when flying. More earthbound birds with webbed feet have a problem when sleeping, because they cannot roost in the safety of trees. In having to sleep on land or water they do so by sleeping in flocks, peeking with one eye open and the other closed—literally keeping an eye out for danger. Ducks on the edge of a sleeping group keep their open eye outwards, and after a while the bird will turn around so that the other eye can take over the watch-keeping. Apparently, a duck can be fooled if it sleeps alone but alongside a mirror, when it thinks that it is sleeping next to a vigilant companion, and it keeps that side's eye closed for much longer than the other. One-eyed sleep is also found in penguins and probably many other bird species, if we did but know it.

Half asleep

Not only can ducks sleep with only one eye shut; the same happens with their brains. Much of what a bird sees in one eye goes to the other side of its brain, which allows it to sleep with the side of the brain connected to the closed eye, while the other side, linked to the peeking eye, can stay awake. Dolphins and at least some other whales have developed this 'half-asleep' technique to a much more sophisticated degree, and can certainly sleep with one side of the brain, while the other remains awake.[5] After an hour or so like this, the roles switch over, with the sleeping side waking up and the other side going to sleep. Similar to ducks, dolphins sleep with one eye open and the other closed, and this tends to reflect which side of the brain happens to be sleeping, with the closed eye being on the opposite side to the sleeping half of the brain. If the animal is only in light sleep, then both sides of the brain can doze together. By the way, in humans, vision from both eyes goes to both sides of the brain, which prevents us from having this 'half sleep'.

The probable reason for dolphin half sleep is not so much to do with the dangers of sleeping in the open sea (as they have few enemies), but because they have to continue swimming while sleeping, so that they can surface and breathe. Dolphins must keep surfacing every few minutes for air, unlike some of their larger cousins, such as sperm whales, which are able to dive to great depths and hold their breath for long periods. The most studied animal in this respect is the 'bottle-nose' dolphin. During sleep these dolphins slowly spiral up to the surface in a characteristic and usually counter-clockwise way, breathe and then sink back down. Another astonishing discovery with this animal is that it has no rapid eye movement or REM (dreaming) sleep at all.[5,6] We do not know whether this may have anything to do with potential problems linked to dreaming, because the confusion in having half one's brain dreaming and the other awake would be bewildering, to say the least.

Each side of the dolphin's brain can be sleep deprived separately,[4] simply by waking the animal up as soon as this side sleeps, while letting the other side sleep normally. The side allowed to sleep does not sleep longer to compensate for the lost sleep on the other side. Instead, when the animal sleeps with the deprived side, there is usually a large sleep 'rebound', with more deep sleep than for the non-deprived side. However, some dolphins show no rebound at all,[5,6] which is another extraordinary finding.

Another type of dolphin has a different sleep peculiarity. The 'blind Indus dolphin' lives in the shallow and turbid estuarine waters of the Indus river. It swims on its side and has lost the use of its eyes (the water is too muddy to see through), although it has a very good sonar system. Incredibly, it virtually never really stops swimming, seemingly because of the dangerous environment in which it lives, especially during the monsoon when the Indus floods, sweeping along uprooted trees and other debris. The animal has to be very alert, not only avoiding these rapidly moving objects, but also avoiding being dashed against the rocks below. Cessation of swimming for more than just a moment would leave it vulnerable to being swept along by the current, and injury. Sleeping with one side of the brain will not work here, because swimming has to be vigorous and cannot be maintained to a sufficient degree in sleep. So, this dolphin sleeps for around a minute at a time, taking hundreds of these 'microsleeps' each day. During a microsleep, swimming slows down but does not cease. When all the microsleeps are added up they come to about seven hours a day.

The remarkable adaptations to the sleep patterns of these dolphins must point to sleep serving a vital purpose, otherwise it is difficult to imagine why they retain sleep at all, rather than not lose it during evolution—as happened with the Indus dolphin's useless eyes.

The fur seal, like the bottle-nosed dolphin, has a similar 'half-brain' sleeping habit when at sea.[5,6] Here, it sleeps on its side, under the surface with its nostrils just out of the water. The flipper in the water is controlled by the awake side of the brain, and gently moves to stabilise the animal. The other flipper, operated by the sleeping side of the brain, rests alongside the body. After an hour or so, the roles reverse and the animal flips its body over. When at sea, which can be for months at a time, the fur seal also has no REM sleep, maybe for reasons similar to the bottle-nosed dolphin. Although REM sleep reappears when the seal sleeps on land, there is no compensatory increase in this type of sleep to make up for what was lost at sea. This rather surprising finding in such intelligent animals, including dolphins, certainly questions the importance of REM sleep.

Much of the credit for these remarkable findings with dolphins and seals goes to Professor Lev Mukhametov, working in Russia, and more recently to Professors Oleg Lyamin and Jerry Siegel in Los Angeles. Their most recent finding is probably the most extraordinary of all, and concerns newborn killer whales and dolphins.[7] These youngsters seem not to sleep at all for the first three weeks or more of their lives because, for safety, they have to stay in continuous physical contact with the mother—who does not sleep either—but for only the first two weeks! The two eyes of both the mother and the newborn remain open continuously throughout these periods and, furthermore, there seems to be no rebound recovery sleep in either animal afterwards. There is no real explanation of how these animals deal with the apparent sleep loss, especially as both mother and infant seem to thrive, with no sign of any stress or other physical effects. As for their brains, and the seemingly vital role that sleep has for the cortex (more about this later), all I can guess is that, rather than sleep with half the brain at a time, perhaps smaller parts of the brain can somehow go 'off-line' and recover during this prolonged wakefulness.

Fitful sleepers

Bigger animals show that they are asleep, or intend to sleep, by adopting a typical posture—cats curl up and horses lie with their heads alongside their flanks. Easily done, whereas the ungainly giraffe undergoes various laborious contortions, just for sleeping only two hours a night, when, if it wants to obtain anything better than drowsiness or very light sleep, it has to get down on its haunches. The problem is not so much with lying down, but in getting up again, because this takes about 15 seconds, which is a long time if there is danger around. The giraffe never sleeps like this for more than an hour at a time, and maybe only for 20 minutes. So, it has to get down and stand up several times a night, to obtain its 'quality sleep'. For the rest of the night it stands drowsily, propped against a tree. After getting down on its haunches, it sits with its neck vertical for a few minutes, checking for safety and chewing the cud. When sleep ensues, its neck sags into an 'S' shape, chewing ceases, and the eyes stay open but unfocused. Periodically during this sleep, its neck and head sag further to lie along the flank in a 'sleeping swan' position, and the eyes are closed; this is probably REM sleep, but lasts for only a few minutes at a time.

Sleep is a vulnerable state to be in unless you happen to be very safe, particularly if you are large or have no enemies or predators, such as the elephant, lion and gorilla. To the question, 'where and for how long does a gorilla sleep?' the answer is simply 'wherever and for as long as it wants to'. The record for the longest sleeper goes to the South American two-toed sloth, which spends around 20 hours asleep per day, up in the highest branches of the rain forests out of sight, and certainly out of the mind of any predator. On the other hand, antelope are fitful sleepers, sleeping in herds, with only those individuals in the centre able to sleep safely. Being on the herd's perimeter means either no sleep or becoming someone's dinner. For those on the outside, the trick is to creep into the centre of the herd and let those who have slept peacefully take over guard duties. Watching these herds at night, one can see this fascinating herding movement. Flocks of sheep also do this at night, but to a lesser extent, perhaps because they feel safer than antelope.

Sheep kept in pens, horses in stables, or cows in barns all sleep longer than when in the field, perhaps knowing that they are safer indoors. Pet cats sleep longer when well fed and kept indoors, than when out hunting for their supper. Whether this longer sleep is also because of boredom, or feeling safer, is a matter for debate—probably both. But the real question is, 'since they sleep less in the wild, are they sleep deprived, or are they simply sleeping to an unnecessary excess when confined?'. If antelope, sheep, and other vulnerable animals were so sleepy in the wild, then this would not be safe if there were predators around. It is more likely, I suspect, that when they feel safe, in a restricted space, they simply take more sleep than they actually need—which is a hot topic when it comes to human sleep (see Chapter 18).

For one reason or another, all animals have to sleep, and there are no permanent non-sleepers, even among those living in the most dangerous conditions—which all points to sleep having essential life-preserving purposes. With mammals, the reasons for sleep probably differ somewhat, depending on their body size and the complexity of their brains—in other words, the reasons why we humans need to sleep must be subtly different from those of the mouse, for example.

The great immobiliser

Small mammals, like mice, must eat huge amounts of food to fuel the metabolic fire that keeps them alive. Their predicament is that because of their small size they lose a great deal of their heat through their skin and extremities, which they have to make up by producing more heat from the digestion and metabolism of their food. Although their hair or fur offers some insulation, it cannot be too thick, otherwise they could not move, other than just to roll around! To understand their problem, imagine a cube-shaped mouse with its six sides—each side loses body heat to the outside. Double the size of the mouse by putting two mice together, and two of the six surfaces of each mouse lie against each other and will not lose so much heat—in effect this bigger mouse has 10 not 12 sides. Double this size again into a giant mouse—maybe to the size of a rat—and 6 more sides are protected in this way, with only 16 of the 24 sides exposed, and so on. So the bigger the mammal the smaller relatively is its surface area, and the less it has to worry about heat loss. Moreover, the less this heat loss, the less food has to be eaten to provide fuel for its 'body fire'. Whereas a well-fed human can go without food for many days and survive quite well, apart from losing some weight (mainly fat), a starved mouse will live only a day or so, because it loses so much heat that cannot adequately be replenished. The starved rat, being larger, will last out maybe a week. As body heat comes from the calories in food, the mouse has to eat huge amounts—maybe half its body weight each day. This is why so much of its wakefulness has to be spent not only in foraging and feeding to make up for its heat loss, but also in grooming its fur to ensure that it retains its heat-insulating properties. When all this is done, it sleeps—and that is what life is all about for the mouse: eat, sleep, groom, and, for the female, rear infants.

How does all this relate to sleep? It makes mice huddle together to form a 'giant mouse', reducing their heat loss and saving huge amounts of energy, especially when they're in a well-insulated nest. For example, when four mice are huddled together, their total heat loss is half that of four separate animals—the more in a huddle, the better! Sadly, as some might say, such huddling is not really for humans because for our large bodies this simply means that, collectively, we will usually overheat! Sleep has another energy-saving benefit for mice and other small mammals, because it also stops them from needlessly running around and wasting energy, that is sleep provides them with the only real opportunity for physical rest—it is their 'great immobiliser'. Better still, for some small mammals such as the North American ground squirrel, sleep can also develop into a 'torpor', whereby the animal's body temperature falls way below its normal level for a few hours during sleep. This process provides more energy saving because there is no need to produce, or lose, so much body heat.

Torpor, by the way, is not a minor form of hibernation—the two are quite distinct. Hibernation is a prolonged period, lasting weeks or months, when body temperature falls even further, sometimes down to a few degrees above freezing. It is mostly found in small mammals living in very cold climates, where food is scarce in the winter. Hibernation provides huge energy savings and is the only way some small mammals can survive the winter. Hibernation is not a profound form of sleep, as is commonly thought, because hibernating mammals still have to arouse from hibernation in order to obtain some sleep. This is one of the fascinating findings about hibernators because, to go to sleep, they have to raise their body temperature, which is a lengthy and laborious process taking many hours. The brain has to be fairly warm in order to sleep and, having slept, the animal slips back into hibernation. Seemingly, the need for sleep accumulates during hibernation, but more slowly than usual, and has to be paid off after this laborious arousal process, which is so costly in energy terms. It further points to sleep having vital, life-sustaining roles, especially for the brain.

For the mouse and its relatives there is no time for sitting and relaxing outside the nest—too dangerous in any case. Besides, they do not have the capacity for relaxed wakefulness anyway. Surprisingly, relaxation is not just an absence of behaviour, but an advanced activity requiring a particularly intricate brain, which the mouse does not have. Relaxed wakefulness is a highly evolved, complex behaviour and not simply being in a 'zombie-like' state with a blank mind, thinking and doing nothing. It usually involves watching something with interest, maybe contemplating about where the next meal is coming from, or just pondering about life in general. For us, it usually involves reading, talking, listening, and watching—even the TV. This relaxed wakefulness is more typical of larger mammals—not that they watch TV or read newspapers, but that they are more prepared and able to sit, watch, and listen. It is as if their minds are preoccupied. Maybe they do have time to 'while away', because their relatively large bodies mean that they need relatively less food and do not have to spend so much time, as the mouse does, in looking for food and eating.

I'm being unashamedly anthropomorphic here—attributing

human characteristics to these larger animals, such as the dog and cat—but why not? Their brains are more advanced and much better developed than those of rodents. Even the most 'intelligent' rodent cannot do these things. Seemingly, it cannot sit and do nothing—it has to do something—and this invariably involves physical activity of one sort or another—grooming, foraging, eating, etc.

For humans, other apes, monkeys, and advanced mammals such as dogs, cats, sheep, cows, horses, and just about all other hoofed mammals, sleep is no longer the 'great immobiliser'. They can all lie awake relaxed but vigilant, because their well-developed brains allow them to do this. This ability to rest during wakefulness, together with the larger body size, means that sleep no longer provides big energy savings. Take us, for example—rather than sleep for eight hours overnight, if we sat relaxed and read a book instead (assuming that we could stay awake), then the small further increase in energy saved by sleeping rather than resting like this is equivalent to only the calories provided by a slice of bread or a handful of peanuts—a meagre reason for sleeping! Moreover, given the vulnerability of those larger mammals that are not safe when asleep, there must be more to sleep than mere immobility and energy conservation, which is the basis for sleep in small mammals. Put simply, whereas for us sleep is not particularly important as an energy conserver, for the mouse it most certainly is. On the other hand, sleep seems to be much more vital to our more advanced brain.

Stress

Depriving an animal of sleep is the obvious way of finding out what sleep is really doing for it. This sounds easy, but the problem with animals is that the methods for keeping them awake can be more stressful and damaging than the sleep loss itself. The most studied animal in this respect is the laboratory rat—even though it is a rather unusual rat, being albino and very inbred. The most impressive studies of sleep deprivation in this animal were carried out by Dr Allan Rechtschaffen and his team, at the Chicago University Sleep Research Laboratory.[8] They used a sophisticated piece of apparatus whereby two rats each sat on their half of a large circular platform, separated by a vertical divide, with the whole platform surrounded by water. One of the pair was sleep deprived and the other, a 'yoked control' animal, could snatch sleep. In theory, both endured the same degree of general stress (exposed on a rotating platform surrounded by water, etc.), whereas the control animal was not so sleep deprived as its less fortunate partner. Thus, any greater effect with the sleep-deprived animal was attributed to the extra sleep loss. Whenever the totally sleep-deprived animal attempted to sleep, the platform rotated and, if it did not get up and move in the opposite direction of the rotation, it was gently shunted into the water. Rats hate getting wet and will avoid a dunking at almost any cost. The control rat on the other side of the platform had to move at the same time, whether it was asleep or awake, otherwise it would also get a dipping. Nevertheless, it was able to sleep for as long as its hapless companion remained awake, when the platform would remain stationary, only to move when this animal began nodding off.

This is a very effective method of totally depriving the rat of sleep, although the animal inevitably falls into the water on occasions, unlike its somewhat drier and perhaps less unhappy companion. It certainly becomes more bedraggled and seems to give up grooming its fur. This is a vital activity for rats and other rodents, as it helps keep them insulated from excessive heat loss. The sleep deprived rat also loses precious body heat from its large and exposed tail. Seemingly, to make up for this heat loss it eats voraciously—which is not sufficient, because it eventually loses weight through the disappearance of its body fat and other energy reserves. After about two weeks of this regimen, the totally sleep-deprived rat's body temperature falls to a critically low level, the animal develops blood poisoning (septicaemia), and it dies. By this time the control animal is less bedraggled and in a healthier, although not healthy, state. Remarkably, if the totally sleep-deprived animal is allowed to sleep almost at this end-point, it will rapidly and fully recover. The Chicago scientists believed that death in these animals is linked to the body heat loss running out of control, whereas Dr Carol Eversen, from the University of Wisconsin, believes the septicaemia to be the fatal factor, linked to a failure of the immune system and collapse of all resistance to disease.

Moreover, she thinks that it is likely that the early stages of septicaemia may underlie the initial fall in both body weight and temperature (infections in rats do not usually cause a fever—often the opposite). The immune system is enormously complex, with so many different facets, even in the rat. Sleep or the lack of it may well have a subtle effect here, but we have yet to find out what might really be going on.

Postmortem examinations on the sleep-deprived rats show no diseased organs, apart from skin sores. Nevertheless, both the sleep-deprived and the control animals are stressed by the experience, because the levels of the hormone, cortisol, which helps them (as well as us) to cope with stress, is produced in similar, large amounts in both animals. On the face of it, this suggests that both animals were equally stressed, and that the sleep-deprived animal died because of the sleep deprivation rather than any extra stress. Another possibility is that cortisol and other body defences utilised by both animals to cope with the stresses reached maximum levels, which were sufficient for the control animal to survive, but insufficient to stop the sleep-deprived rat from dying, because it was even more stressed from being more bedraggled, etc. What, I think, is impressive here is not so much that the sleep-deprived rats died, but that they lived for so long (a fortnight or so) under these arduous conditions. Bearing in mind that the normal life expectancy for a rat is only around two years, on this rather loose argument, two weeks in a rat's life is a relatively lengthy period.

Cortisol protects the body against excess damage during stressing situations, especially by reducing inflammation of one sort or another. It is why we use a synthetic form of cortisol (cortisone), in moderation, for reducing joint and skin inflammation. Unfortunately, cortisol is a two-edged sword because it can also suppress the body's ability to fight off infection. Cortisol is released into our blood, from glands above the kidneys, in small amounts throughout the day, especially around 6am, probably in anticipation of the greater pressures from the waking day. Levels rise further whenever we are put under physical or mental strain—not only from an injury, but also, for example, during stressful, competitive exercise and when we are exposed to uncomfortably hot or cold environments. Probably the greatest cause of cortisol output for us comes from our state of mind, such as apprehension and fear. These are very potent triggers for its release; this psychological factor is more powerful than any other and must not be underestimated.

Fear may be one reason why the sleep-deprived rat seems to suffer so badly. It contrasts with sleep-deprived human volunteers who seem to cope well by comparison. Without sleep, we can be very sleepy and irritable, but provided that we know that no harm will come to us and that we can withdraw from the experiment whenever we like, the deprivation will not necessarily be stressful. On the other hand, sleep-deprived rats are not volunteers and have no insight into what is happening. I'm speculating, here, of course, as to whether the raised cortisol levels in these rats is caused by illness, fear alone, fear caused by the illness, or whatever.

Interestingly, these sleep-deprived animals show no signs of diabetes, which contrasts with recent claims that even short-term sleep loss in humans is harmful, causing problems in the way that the body handles sugars ('glucose intolerance'), and leading to what might seem to be a 'pre-diabetic' state. I deal with this topic in Chapter 18.

Although 'pure sleep deprivation' in humans may not be very stressful, this assumption is based on otherwise undemanding and fairly pleasant laboratory studies, which are not very realistic, because in the real world people are often sleep deprived as a result of other stresses such as long and arduous working hours, or family crises. Such stresses, alone, will raise cortisol levels. Even worrying about the sleep loss itself, and whether we will be able to cope with it, will increase cortisol output—a clear case of 'mind over matter'. People with insomnia, by the way, often have high cortisol levels, which they may well attribute to the apparent lack of sleep. It is more probable, however, that this is caused by other reasons that lead to both the cortisol rise and the poor sleep (see Chapter 19).

Healthy people who volunteer for sleep deprivation experiments are usually well cosseted by their experimenters, perhaps too much so, and may be inadvertently protected from the full effects of sleep loss. Apart from the sleep deprivation, volunteers typically lead a tranquil existence, are fed very well, and, except for having periodically to undergo various tests, have plenty of time for relaxation, reading, and watching TV. There have been many of these experiments with human volunteers, with the longest lasting 11 days, as will be seen shortly. Surprisingly, the physical effects of this sleep loss in humans are conspicuous by their absence—there is just a general slowing up of most body functions, with only a trivial fall of body temperature (about 0.5°C) and no weight loss. We also show a rise in the number of white blood cells in the blood, although this seems to be within normal limits and not of great clinical concern. For us, however, it is not so much the body that is affected by sleep loss, but the cerebral cortex and our behaviour, as we will see.

More extreme studies of human sleep deprivation have been run by military research groups, in enterprises referred to by the military as 'sustained operations'—SUSOPs for short. Here, some of the ethical and safety factors required for the civilian volunteer can be put aside, and, typically, sleep loss is for three days of continuously simulated battle, including heavy exercise, food restriction, competition, and other stresses. Not surprisingly, the outcome for the soldier is more eventful, but not serious. Again we do not know to what extent these effects are caused by sleep loss or the other factors, because, unlike the civilians in the laboratory, who can pull out of the experiment whenever they want to, the soldier cannot do this and has to cope somehow. Anxiety about what may happen to them, whether they can cope, and how they will live up to the expectations of their comrades will all add to the soldier's stress and, not surprisingly, cause a large rise in cortisol levels.

One of the earliest accounts of SUSOPs comes from a junior officer with Ulpius Marcellus, governor of Britannia from AD 180 to 184, who was also known as 'the Wakeful One'. During his vigorous campaigns into southern Scotland, he showed himself to be more wakeful than any other general. As he wanted everyone else to know this, and for all his commanders to be alert as well, he would write orders on wooden tablets, almost every evening, and send an aide to deliver these to his officers at various hours during the night, so that they believed him to be always awake. Worse still, they were expected to be awake in order to receive and respond accordingly. As he advocated fasting as a method for remaining awake, one can only imagine what sort of fighting condition his officers were in, and it is not surprising that his army never succeeded in conquering any part of Scotland. Needless to say, Marcellus was a cause of much of the unrest sweeping through the Roman army in Britain at the time, and he was recalled to Rome.

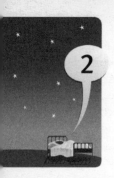

2 By the brain, for the brain

Brain strain

What is going on in the mind of my cat, sitting on the windowsill for the last half an hour, attentively watching the birds on the lawn, or in the mind of my dog lying there in its basket with ears pricked up and following my every move? Probably, uncharitable thoughts towards birds in the case of the cat and fun and games for the dog. Or, to be more serious, let us call it 'quiet readiness'. It is a characteristic of a fairly advanced brain, which both these animals do have. Even when sitting relaxed like this, their brains are alert, busy, and ready for action. Intently watching something happen, especially if the scene is changing from moment to moment, and a quick response is required, puts quite a demand on the brain, whether it be that of a dog, cat, or human. This is what 'brain work' is really about, and can easily involve the active engagement of most of the high level centres of the brain, that is, much of the entire cerebral cortex. Quiet readiness can create a greater workload for the cortex than that produced by reading, solving a crossword, or even playing a game of chess. Although these last two tasks seem to 'strain the brain', only small areas of cortex are really 'strained', whereas intently watching, listening to, and otherwise sensing something in the wider environment that is attention grabbing mobilise much more of the cortex.

The cortex can be likened to the canopy of a mushroom, with the stem underneath containing the controls for vital body functions and simple behaviours. All mammals have a similar brain stem because we all have similar needs for the control of basic body functions. On the other hand, it is the cortex that becomes relatively larger in the advanced mammals, culminating with humans. An increasingly large cortex causes it to become crumpled, or 'convoluted', rather like the surface of a shelled walnut. The larger and more convoluted it is, the more complex the behaviour that can be produced. Our cortex is the most complex and crumpled of all, so much so that it almost completely envelops the brain stem, as in a 'button mushroom' where the stem is hidden from view. In contrast, 'simpler' mammals such as mice have a relatively smooth, rather small cortex that does not envelop the brain stem, as in a flat-topped mushroom where the stem is clearly seen. Most mammals, especially those larger than a rabbit, have a cortex with at least some convolution. The dog and cat are fairly well endowed in this respect, as are their wild relatives and hoofed and cloven-footed mammals, including sheep, which, technically at least, are not as stupid as commonly thought. All these animals display relaxed wakefulness with quiet readiness, although, as a general rule, those that hunt prey have an even more advanced cortex and a greater repertoire of behaviour than a similarly sized mammal that stares at and eats grass all day.

Unlike the rest of the body, the cortex cannot really relax during wakefulness, because it is worked hard, even in 'quiet readiness'. When we lie relaxed on a comfortable bed, in a darkened sound-proof room, with eyes closed, ears plugged, without a care in the world, and the mind cleared of all thoughts, our cortex remains in quiet readiness. This also applies to various waking meditative states because, despite what might be claimed to the contrary, the cortex still cannot relax. The only time our cortex can really rest and recover to any extent is during sleep, which is why sleep loss mostly affects our cortex and behaviour, as will be seen later. As mammals go, the more complex the cortex, the more important sleep is for brain recovery from its waking workload. It so happens that a more sophisticated cortex tends to be found in larger mammals. A larger body allows more 'free time' from eating, which, in turn, provides for more relaxed wakefulness, when the body can recover without necessitating sleep.

Let me re-cap by turning this argument around—the smaller the mammal, the more it has to eat and spend time in feeding. There is little or no 'spare' time for relaxed wakefulness, which a small mammal cannot display anyway, because its brain is too poorly developed to produce this behaviour. Although its sleep allows for brain recovery, sleep is really for immobility and saving energy. In sum, the evolution of mammals has brought a subtle change to sleep, from being mostly an energy conserver to providing recovery for the increasingly complex cortex.

Sleeping like a baby

Infancy for all mammals is the time of life when the cortex works particularly hard, with huge amounts of waking brain work resulting from so many new experiences, and when the cortex has to make so many new connections within its myriad cells. For all mammals, the waking infant cortex is designed to learn particularly fast, because it is 'plastic' and malleable to new experiences. Sleep plays a particularly important role here, as it is thought that many of these new connections take place during sleep. With ageing, this plasticity slows up and, literally, it is difficult to teach an old dog new tricks—although, fortunately, this is not so much the case with old humans, as we will see. Nevertheless, it does mean that, for most mammals, the role of sleep in cortical recovery diminishes somewhat over the lifespan. We are, however, unique in this respect, because our adult brain retains much of this plasticity, as shown by our ability to continue learning up to a ripe old age. Admittedly, this declines somewhat as we get older, but to nothing like the extent found in other mammals. More fascinating is that we adults retain many more infant-like behaviours that are usually lost in other adult mammals. I do not mean that human adults are childish and immature, but, rather, that we retain into adulthood a high degree of learning ability, curiosity, exploration, and playfulness—behaviours similar to those of the infant. From the perspective that sleep provides the cortex with the ability for these plastic and other learning processes to recover from the activities of wakefulness, our sleep probably does not change that much from infancy to adulthood, as it does in other mammals when these processes slow up.

Indeed, we adults are remarkably child like. Although we get larger, our overall appearance does not, of course, change that much when it is compared with our nearest relative, the chimpanzee. Take a look at the picture of the baby chimpanzee's head in comparison with its mum in Figure 1. Whereas junior's face is fairly small compared with the rest of his head, especially his cranium (brain case), for mum it is the reverse, with her prominent face and snout dominating her head. Contrast their eyebrow ridges, foreheads, and the angle that the head makes with the back. Even more captivating is how junior looks more like us than his mum, and how similar he looks to both the infant and the adult human. Or, put differently, we are just overgrown infants! This similarity is seen throughout much of the human body, right down to the feet, as Figure 2 shows, which compares the feet from the human baby and adult with those of a macaque monkey. Of the four feet, the odd one out is clearly that of the adult monkey (look at the position of its big toe compared with those in the other feet)—these other feet are very similar to each other. To get to the point, the same

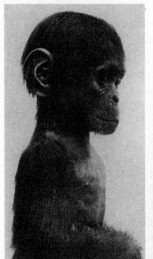
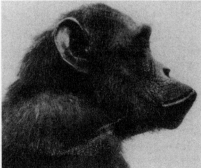

Figure 1 The infant chimp looks more like us than its mum. Baby and adult chimpanzees from Naef,[1] who remarks: 'Of all animal pictures known to me, this is the most manlike' (p 118).

Monkey Human

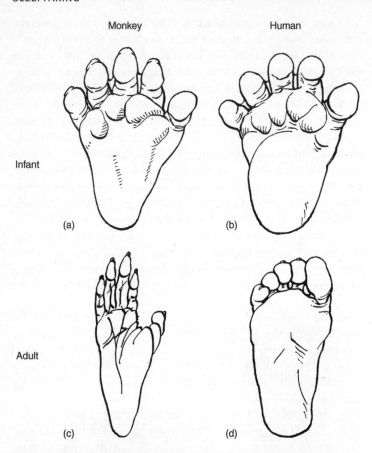

Infant

(a) (b)

Adult

(c) (d)

Figure 2 Which is the odd one out? (a and c) Feet are from baby and adult Macaque monkeys; (b and d) feet from a human newborn baby and an adult. (From de Beer,[2] reproduced by permission of Oxford University Press.)

applies to the shape of the infant and adult human cortex, as both also resemble that of the infant monkey and ape, much more so than that of the adult ape. So, I argue, the same applies to our sleep—its role for our cortex changes less with age than it does for other apes, monkeys, and probably all other mammals for that matter. So we do, indeed, sleep like a baby!

Memory

'Brain plasticity' covers a multitude of activities, with learning being only one aspect. In broad terms brain plasticity deals with the ability to react appropriately to change, and to adapt to and deal with new information from our surroundings. It is knowledge: knowing what to do and what not to do, especially during new encounters, and utilising previous experiences. The speed by which we adapt to change is also a central feature of 'plasticity'. Meeting new people, places, and things, and being able to assimilate and deal with all the new sensory experiences coming in at once from the eyes, ears, nose, and hands, together place a huge waking demand on the brain and especially the cortex. This is just a more elaborate explanation of the 'brain work' mentioned earlier. In providing recovery from this bombardment, sleep probably allows the cortex to make appropriate adjustments—that is, the adjustments involving 'plastic processes', which encompass learning and the formation of memories.

Laboratory studies of how the brain forms memories usually depend on very simple tasks, reflecting only small and often unusual aspects of human behaviour. Even so, how exactly these learning and memory events produce changes in the brain are still poorly understood, let alone how sleep may help these processes. Roughly speaking, learning and memory can be divided into two broad areas: first, the conscious memorising of facts and information, which is called 'declarative learning', for example, writing down and telling others what we have learnt (this new information is consciously stated [that is, 'declared']); second, the 'procedural learning' of skills, such as riding a bike, driving a car, playing darts, swimming, which are subconscious, because they usually defy explanation in words, and are simply a matter of 'practice makes perfect'. Whereas procedural learning is easily seen in animals, the heavy reliance of declarative learning on language means that it can really be studied only in humans.

Research into how sleep affects procedural learning has mostly been with animals, using simple laboratory tasks that may or may not have relevance to the animal's natural behaviour. None of the findings into the potentially beneficial effects of sleep on procedural learning have been dramatic, but there is something happening. Even though rapid eye movement (REM) sleep (see Chapter 14) has been linked to procedural learning, REM sleep is not essential for it, at least in the human adult.[3] However, we do not really know what happens in the infant, because little or no appropriate research has been done.

The ability to learn and memorise anything clearly depends on being awake and alert. Nevertheless, declarative learning in human adults seems to benefit from the deep form of non-REM (NREM) sleep (see Chapter 13), although, again, only simple tasks have been used to demonstrate this effect. Memorising a new experience is certainly influenced by what happens immediately after the event, because the formation of the memory will be interfered with if something interesting and distracting appears soon afterwards. On the other hand, ensuing sleep will minimise this interference and recall may be improved after sleep for this reason alone, rather than sleep providing some sort of memory 'glue'. Obviously, sleep is quite different from wakefulness, and possibly the more unlike the ensuing activity is from the event to be remembered, the less likely it is that the memory formation will be interfered with. Thus, learning experiences followed by waking activities that are more similar to the original learning than to sleep are not remembered so well. I am playing devil's advocate here, because I do suspect that sleep does something beneficial to declarative memory. However, the excellent studies that have shown this so far with humans have not demonstrated profound effects of sleep, but rather smaller, albeit statistically significant, improvements.

Another mystery is how the brain knits together the sensations from the eyes, ears, and other senses experienced in everyday life, to produce memories of the whole scene. How are we able to see a picture of someone's face and then recall not the related visual memories, but memories from another sense—for example, what that person may have said? Or identify an odour or touch an object and then recall a whole series of related visual and emotional events? Whether and how sleep may help with the sorting out and connecting up of these more complex but commonplace memories have yet to be discovered, and are one of the more exciting routes for sleep research to take. How perceptive was Shakespeare with Macbeth's renowned remark that sleep 'knits up the ravell'd sleave of care'? A *sleave*, by the way, is a knotted ball of unspun silk.

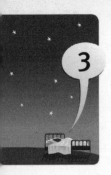

3 The substance of sleep

Guts of the matter

Apart from believing sleep to be some sort of recovery process, most early ideas looked only at how sleep might be brought about, rather than at what it really does. The two approaches can be quite different. For example, aperitifs and the smell and sight of food all promote eating but they do not explain why we eat. Even after a filling meal, these stimuli can tempt us to eat more, but this extra food is unnecessary for our well-being or waistlines! Most early civilisations thought sleep was due to something that built up in the brain during wakefulness and dissipated during sleep. Aristotle[1] thought along these lines 2000 years ago, and proposed that sleep resulted from warm vapours rising from within the stomach:

> The evaporation attendant upon the process of nutrition. . . . naturally tends to move upward. This explains why fits of drowsiness are especially apt to come after meals. It also follows certain forms of fatigue; for fatigue operates as a solvent, and the dissolved [warm] matter acts like food prior to digestion.

The beginning of the twentieth century also produced many of what are termed 'humoral' theories, whereby various sleep-inducing substances were supposed to accumulate in the brain. These ranged from known chemicals such as lactic acid, carbon dioxide, and cholesterol, to the vaguely described 'leucomaines' and 'urotoxins', whatever these were. Nevertheless, by 1907 some progress had been made when two French researchers, Dr Rene Legendre and Dr Henri Pieron,[2] claimed to have found a substance, which they called 'hypnotoxin', in sleep-deprived animals. This was a great boost to the protagonists of the humoral theories, particularly those coming from Germany, where there were claims of other new substances such as '*Schlafstoff*' and '*Bromhormon*'. However, real success was hard to come by and interest dwindled—that is, until the 1960s. Great headway has since been made into 'sleep substances', which are now known to influence sleep and its timing, although they are not necessarily the reason why we sleep.

The pioneering work was by Dr John Pappenheimer, in the 1960s, at Harvard Medical School, and subsequently by his protégé Dr Jim Krueger, now at Washington State University. In one of his famous experiments, Pappenheimer sleep deprived goats and discovered a then unknown substance, named 'factor S', in their cerebrospinal fluid. When given to other animals it readily produced sleep. Factor S can be extracted from human urine—3,000 litres of urine being required to produce seven-millionths of a gram of factor S. Nevertheless, this was potent enough to be divided up into 500 doses which, when individually given to rabbits, caused a sleep lasting for about six hours. Surprisingly, they could be woken up mid-sleep, without difficulty, and then might eat or groom for a short while, only to return to sleep.

As factor S is a substance that closely resembles chemicals found in bacteria, it was first thought that it was simply some form of bacterial contamination of the samples taken. But further detective work by Krueger and colleagues[3] found that, although it may well have come originally from the remains of bacteria in the gut and lungs, and been destroyed by the body's defence system, it was then being utilised by the brain as part of its own biochemistry. Indeed, early accounts of the causes of yawning, dating from the Victorians, may have had great prescience in claiming that yawning was caused by 'autointoxication by waste products from bacteria in the bowel'.

Factor S has been synthesised in various forms, and one variety produces excessive amounts of sleep when injected into a variety of mammals—rats, rabbits, cats, and monkeys. Unfortunately it cannot be used as the new wonder drug for insomnia because it takes about three hours to become effective and causes an unwanted fever! As we know, sleepiness often accompanies fever, for example, in influenza. However, Krueger found that it was not so much factor S that caused the fever, but a knock-on effect that stimulated the body's immune system and led to fever. Specifically it was the action of the 'interleukins', a group of substances coming under the collective term of 'cytokines', mostly produced by white blood cells. Krueger further established that it was not the fever itself that caused the sleepiness, because, by giving aspirin to lower the fever, but not the interleukin levels, sleepiness remained.

Essences

Cytokines and interleukins are linked to sleep as well as to a myriad of other body functions. They come in many complex forms, some of which give the immune system a boost. This is not to say that sleep necessarily rejuvenates the immune system because, in contrast, nonstressful sleep deprivation can also boost the immune system, but in another way. There are findings, with animals, that a limited amount of sleep deprivation can even help to regress certain cancers. It could be argued that when asleep we are in a 'low' state, and potentially more vulnerable to infection. Therefore, as a precaution, the immune system is cranked up. Alternatively, in going without sleep we might be exposed to more infections, by encountering more bacteria when moving around more than normal. Thus, another turn of the immune crank is needed. Although the pragmatic answer to all this is that our immune system may simply be adjusting its vast array of defence mechanisms to suit the circumstances, something unknown but subtle may be happening to immunity during sleep.

Krueger's pioneering studies on rabbits have shown that, when they are infected with harmful bacteria, not only do they develop a fever, but they also sleep much longer and deeper than usual. Those doing so to the greatest extent are more likely to survive, which could be seen as sleep benefiting the immune system and its ability to fight off infection. However, there are other alternatives. For example, maybe the shorter sleeping animals were somehow weaker to start with. Serious virus infections in humans do change the structure of our sleep, even when there is no fever. Human immunodeficiency virus (HIV) (without AIDS) is a good example of where sleep changes have been attributed to the greater activity of the body's cytokines. But we cannot be sure that the altered sleep is linked to the immune system trying to fight off viruses, because all that may be happening is that the virus also enters the brain and interferes with the control of sleep itself. Clearly, the interaction between sleep and immunity is a highly complex one.

Apart from all these sleep substances there are numerous other natural chemicals in the brain that influence sleep. 'Neurotransmitters' are the primary way by which nerve cells communicate with each other, and there are several that have a great influence over sleep (and wakefulness), as well as over many body functions and behaviours. The complexity of sleep is further reflected by the many parts of the brain that affect it in one way or another. Some switch sleep on, some switch it off, and others switch off wakefulness—but again, these are not necessarily the real reason for sleep—in the same way that turning on the car's ignition and starting the car up is not the reason for a journey; it is because we want to travel somewhere. We wind up an old-fashioned clock not because we want to see the hands go round, but because we want to know the time. These sleep centres within our brain pave the way for the cortex to progress with its recovery processes during sleep. Other brain centres and brain chemicals influence how sleep is maintained once it has started, and one can liken these to the actual car journey—the journey being sleep. How and when we arrive at our journey's destination (for example, waking up in the morning) depend on many influences: traffic lights, weather conditions, speed limits, road lighting at night, hills, traffic density, whether to take a break, etc. Each can be likened to one of these brain chemicals influencing how sleep proceeds. Inasmuch as traffic density and taking a break not only affect the journey, but also influence other aspects of our behaviour such as irritability, hunger, and thirst, most if not all of these sleep substances and brain chemicals also influence other aspects of our physiology and behaviour, especially eating, drinking, sexual activity, and mood. There is no single 'sleep juice' in the brain that produces sleep and nothing but sleep, and nor is there much prospect for a drug that can substitute for sleep and for all that it does.

Feeding

A possible reason why there seems to be no exclusive sleep substance is because sleep is inextricably tied in with other vital behaviours and physiological needs, especially feeding and how the body controls the use of its energy reserves, and maintains its body temperature. Feeding is linked to sleep by many routes. For example, sleep can stop us feeling hungry, whereas more extreme hunger can prevent sleep and a very large meal can induce sleep. Although sleeping, feeding, drinking, and reproducing may all seem to be quite different behaviours, no two can occur at the same time (with the exception of feeding and drinking), let alone all at once, and it is a matter of give and take. Directly or indirectly, all affect each other and, to return to the topic of brain chemicals and centres, it is efficient for some to have common interests in sleeping, feeding, reproducing, etc., and it makes sense to have common control mechanisms. A good example of a brain substance that affects sleep and other functions is 'orexin–hypocretin'. It was found independently by two groups of scientists, neither of whom were really interested in sleep, but in eating behaviour; each gave it a name derived from Greek, and thus it has its two names: orexin (from *orexis*—to eat) and hypocretin (from the two words *hypo*thalamus [a part of the brain] and 'se*cretin*' [a gut hormone]). It is linked to the control of appetite, metabolism, and obesity and, more interestingly for us, to rapid eye movement (REM) sleep (see Chapter 14).

Orexin–hypocretin also influences another hormone—'leptin'. When our sleep is restricted to around four hours a night, leptin levels fall. Not only does leptin regulate appetite and weight, telling the brain how much energy is available in the body, but in many animals, especially rodents, it also influences reproduction. For us, sleep restriction to four hours also causes a rise in another hormone, 'ghrelin', which makes us want to eat. One explanation for these leptin and ghrelin changes linked to sleep and feeding goes back to our early ancestors, who probably ate more and stored fat during the summer when the days were long and food was plentiful, and who probably slept less at that time of the year. Maybe it was a survival mechanism, preparing the body for the leaner times of the dark winters, when our ancestors had to rely on their body fat and also probably slept for longer.

Stimulants—and coffee houses

As the processes influencing sleep are so complex, and no one drug or even a concoction of drugs is likely to be able to substitute for all the functions of sleep, or eliminate sleepiness for weeks on end, all that can be achieved is to hide some of the effects of sleep loss for a while, especially the feeling of sleepiness. 'Stimulants' do this, with caffeine being the best known. It certainly counteracts the natural brain substance ('adenosine') that accumulates during wakefulness, to promote sleepiness and sleep, and is probably why caffeine reduces or even eliminates sleepiness for a short while, especially if the sleepiness is moderate, as, for example, in the 'afternoon dip' (see Chapter 10).

We all know what sleepiness is, especially what happens during a dull and monotonous task such as motorway driving. However, sleep loss also produces more subtle impairments in the ability to think, which further point to what our sleep is really all about. Caffeine and other stimulants are, up to a point, good at managing sleepiness and improving alertness.[4] Nevertheless, it looks as though these more subtle impairments do not benefit so much from stimulants, and in higher doses these stimulants can enhance the less desirable effects of sleep loss, such as over-confidence, euphoria, risk-taking, and uncharacteristic changes in mood and personality.

Cocaine (from the coca plant) is a powerful stimulant, effective for only about 30 minutes. Although its use is, of course, illegal today, for centuries it was quite socially acceptable, and it was commonly found in tonics and other preparations to allay fatigue. Many of the tales about Sherlock Holmes refer to his resorting to cocaine (albeit against the advice of Dr Watson!). Even the first formulation of Coca-Cola® contained effective amounts of cocaine, which were soon removed, albeit 100 years ago. Amphetamine is another well-known stimulant with similar effects to cocaine, but it lasts much longer, up to six hours, and has been used extensively by the military.[4] Its use has to be strictly controlled, of course, because it is a drug of abuse. Nicotine is also a mild stimulant.

Returning to caffeine, which is mostly found in coffee, many soft drinks, less so in tea, and even in chocolate in small amounts, its stimulating effects have been known for centuries, when the coffee beans just used to be chewed. Roasted and brewed coffee became very popular throughout Europe during the seventeenth century, especially with the establishment in London of 'coffee houses' (nicknamed 'penny universities') when, by 1700, there were around 500 in the capital alone. Whether it was the caffeine that improved alertness and promoted articulated debate in these forerunners to internet cafes, or whether they were simply a convenient venue for the idle rich to gossip and discuss politics, coffee houses had a chequered history of fermenting sedition and were even closed down for a while during the reign of Charles II, 'for disturbing the quiet of the realm'. In London, Samuel Pepys, the famous diarist, used to frequent 'Will's coffee house' (wherever that was), and Samuel Johnson, compiler of the first English dictionary, regularly enjoyed the Turk's Head coffee house on the London Strand, from where much of his inspiration probably came. Beethoven was a reputed coffee drinker, insisting on 60 beans per cup, and Balzac, the French author, claimed that coffee fuelled his writing, which is probably true because there are accounts of his drinking 40 or more cups a day.

Unwittingly or otherwise, most adults in Europe presently consume a minimum of about 200 milligrams of caffeine per day, which is equivalent to about two to three cups of coffee or about eight cups of tea. In the USA, the average daily caffeine consumption can easily double or triple this amount. 'Refreshing' effects, at least to some degree, are usually felt after 20 minutes, lasting from 30 to 90 minutes, depending on how much caffeine is consumed and the extent of the prevailing sleepiness or fatigue. Some people are particularly sensitive to the effects of even small amounts of caffeine, claiming that even one cup of coffee many hours before sleep will lead to a restless night. In contrast, others seem quite resistant and able to consume impressive quantities of coffee in the evening, apparently without any effect on sleep. Whether they have become caffeine 'tolerant' or even caffeine 'dependent' is a somewhat controversial topic. High daily doses of caffeine, beyond about 600 milligrams, can produce agitation, talkativeness, anxiety, and insomnia, as well as heart palpitations and stomach discomfort. On the other hand, cessation of caffeine intake in usually high consumers may bring on symptoms attributed to 'caffeine withdrawal', such as headache, drowsiness, irritability, difficulty in concentrating, and stiffness, appearing within a day. Whether these symptoms were there to begin with, only to be alleviated by caffeine, is a debatable point. I should add that high levels of caffeine were to be found in many 'medicinal tonics' and headache cures, widely available in the USA and Europe 100 or so years ago, where a single dose could easily contain 500 milligrams of caffeine.

It has been claimed that one reason why we apparently consume so much caffeine today is because we live in a sleep-deprived society, and need it as a crutch to overcome endemic daytime sleepiness. However, I suspect that this is largely nonsense because most coffee drinkers simply do it for pleasure and because it is available in so many attractive forms. Nevertheless, as I mentioned, caffeine counteracts the build-up of 'adenosine', a natural brain substance that produces sleep, and in reasonable doses caffeine is effective in dealing with moderate sleepiness. So, the unanswered question remains: what happens to that moderate sleepiness that is knocked out by caffeine— does it reappear later in the day or has it simply vanished? A clue comes from various findings, which show that, if we lose sleep and have the opportunity to make it up, not all of it is recovered (see Chapters 17 and 18), although alertness still returns to normal. It seems that the brain and mind are quite adequately able to deal with some 'missing' sleep without any residual sleepiness. Which brings me on to one of the controversial themes in this book—that there is some spare reserve in the 'average', normal amount of sleep that covers for this contingency. So, for example, if we lose an hour of sleep one night, causing some increased sleepiness that afternoon, then a cup or two of coffee (that is, caffeine) will eliminate this sleepiness and, probably, it will not rebound with a vengeance later that evening.

4 Then

Valiant Gilbert

Nowadays, many of the older studies into human sleep loss, carried out even 30 years ago, are seen to be of only historical interest, dismissed for their antiquity and use of seemingly crude techniques and equipment. Nevertheless, despite the benefits of sophisticated computers in modern times, little has really changed in the outcome from these studies. They are all too easily forgotten—how wrong, because at least one nineteenth-century experiment still remains impressive enough to better many contemporary studies in its standard of science. Ironically, too many of today's sleep scientists undertake what they consider to be cutting edge research, when the answers that they seek are to be found in dusty old tomes stored in library basements.

It is November 1895, at the Iowa University Psychological Laboratory, run by Professor G.T.W. Patrick, who has recently become intrigued by the effects of sleep loss, following his success as a Greek scholar and renowned for his translation of *The Fragments of the Work of Heraclitus of Ephesus on Nature*, which contrasts somewhat with his then just published book, *The Psychology of Profanity*, wherein he gained much of his material by listening to spectators at baseball games. I digress—a preliminary study into sleep loss was called for, to test out some of Patrick's ideas and intended measurements. A volunteer was sought and the unwitting Dr J. Allen Gilbert, Patrick's junior colleague, was recruited. Gilbert was described by Patrick as 'a young man of 28 years, unmarried, of perfect health, of nervous temperament, of very great vitality and activity, who is accustomed to about 8 hours of sound sleep from 10 pm to 6 am' (p 470).[1] Gilbert remained awake continuously for 90 hours, from the night of Wednesday 27 November, to midnight the following Saturday, when he was allowed to sleep. But all was not over as the stoical Gilbert was awoken at hourly intervals to see how deep his sleep was. With much insight Patrick noted that a loud noise would not be practical, here, because the sleeping Gilbert would soon get used to it. So an 'electric garter' was fixed around Gilbert's ankle and the current increased steadily until he awoke to press an 'electric button' by his bedside. The level of the current needed to do this reflected the depth of sleep.

The second hour of his recovery sleep was the deepest, because Gilbert could not be aroused until the current went well beyond expectation, and he 'responded with a cry of pain'—not surprising, as the current was three times greater than what he could tolerate during wakefulness. Eventually he woke spontaneously at 10.30am the next morning, when he later declared himself to be 'wholly refreshed, felt quite as well as ever, and did not feel sleepy the following evening'. The next night he slept for only two extra hours. When the extra sleep taken on these two recovery nights was added together, it came to only a quarter of the total sleep that was lost. To account for this apparent shortfall, Patrick and Gilbert deduced that it was the increased depth of sleep that held the key to recovery—an observation borne out many times since then.

During deprivation Gilbert coped relatively well, although 'on the second night he did not feel well and suffered severely from sleepiness'. The third night he suffered less, and on the fourth day and following evening he felt well and was able to 'pass his time in his usual occupations'. During the final two days he had to be watched closely and could not be left alone because, despite his best efforts, he would fall asleep. Moreover, Patrick noted that 'the daily rhythm was well marked . . . during the afternoon and evening the subject was less troubled with sleepiness. The sleepy period was from midnight until noon, of which the worse part was about dawn' (p 481).[1] How very true.

Gilbert reported having some visual illusions, especially after the second night—for example, 'the floor was covered with a greasy-looking molecular layer of rapidly moving or oscillating particles'. Often this layer was a foot above the floor, which caused him difficulties because he would try to step onto it when walking. Later, the air was full of these dancing particles, apparently developing into swarms of coloured gnats around the gaslight. He even got up on a chair in an attempt to swat them away. Fortunately, these experiences soon disappeared after his recovery sleep.

Systematically, every six hours during the deprivation, and once after the first recovery sleep, Gilbert was given a two-hour series of fourteen psychological tests. As repetition improves performance ('practice makes perfect'), he had to practise these tests thoroughly beforehand, otherwise any deterioration with sleep loss would be counteracted by the improvement with practice. Any net effect of no change might lead to the conclusion that nothing happens with sleep loss. This prior training was a prudent move by Patrick, because even some recent sleep deprivation studies have overlooked this problem. The extent and variety of this testing of Gilbert are impressive even by today's standards, and also included: body temperature and heart rate, body weight, grip and pull strengths, and the average of 15 reaction time responses to 'click' sounds using a Morse-code key, with the subtlety that Gilbert had to respond only to loud clicks and not to soft ones. This was very innovative because it also measures what psychologists nowadays call 'vigilance', and is a technique that provides an extra-sensitive index of sleepiness, which only really came into its own around 70 years later.

Patrick's other measurements were also remarkably astute. Muscle fatigue was assessed from the decline in finger tapping over a minute, and sensitivity to pain was determined by increasing pressure on the fingertip using a 'specially prepared alogmeter' (whatever that was), and 'acuteness of vision', by reading with a candle placed 25 centimetres away.

He paid special attention to several of the findings. Gilbert's body weight increased by 27 ounces (0.8 kg) over the deprivation, and then, perplexingly fell 38 oz (1.1 kg) during the first recovery sleep (we now know that sweating increases during sleep, which would have accounted for some of the weight loss, but not all of it). His grip-and-pull strength weakened, but when the end of the deprivation was in sight he regained his strength (probably because he applied more effort). Reaction time worsened, to return to normal after the first night of sleep. All this may seem unexciting nowadays, but 110 years ago it was the first accurate account of such changes.

Promoted to the status of fellow experimenter for his forbearance, Gilbert joined Patrick to conduct another study on two other volunteers, described as young men 'accustomed to 8–9 hours sound sleep', who underwent 90 hours of sleep deprivation. Neither apparently experienced any illness, hallucinations, or discomfort throughout the proceedings. One had more trouble keeping awake than the other (that is, people vary in the effects of sleep loss) and could not have gone on beyond the 90 hours. Jogging in the streets was good for livening up one of them, especially during the 5am sleepy period. On the first recovery night both slept from 11.15pm to 10.30am the next morning, and this time their sleep was not interrupted by electric shocks, like poor old Gilbert's. They then dozed, one for a further 45 minutes and the other for 4 hours. Surprisingly, it was the person who had coped better during the deprivation who slept for longer. Both then declared that they felt quite refreshed. Despite losing three nights' sleep only one recovery sleep, around 12 hours long, seemed enough for full recovery. Such a small return of lost sleep endorsed the earlier findings of Gilbert.

During the deprivation, similar measurements were made as before, with the addition of tests for remembering shapes, speed in reading letters backwards, and discrimination between two sounds. Even their urine was analysed, for nitrogen and phosphoric acid, with both substances increasing. Patrick and Gilbert could not explain this, but we know now that the most likely reason was that their participants simply ate more food, including protein, which produces this nitrogen. The memory test caused problems for one of them, who became thoroughly confused at one point. The reaction times, and addition and letter-reading tasks were seriously impaired. Inevitably both participants were seen to have frequent very short 'naps' lasting for only seconds, which are nowadays called 'microsleeps' or 'lapses' (see Chapter 7). Daydreaming was frequent. Several times the investigators noted that, if more effort and enthusiasm were put into various tasks, sleepiness could be counteracted for a while, at least until about 60 hours of deprivation. This 60-hour endurance point has been confirmed many times since then. Last, but far from least, Patrick and

Gilbert noticed that the body temperature had fallen about 0.3°C in both people during deprivation, but that its daily rhythm remained. Clearly, they knew of the 24-hour body clock and, again, these findings are the same as reported nowadays.

Surprisingly, both Patrick and Gilbert soon lost interest in the topic of sleep and sleep loss, with Patrick returning to his interests in profanity and producing, in 1913, another book, *Why We Like [American] Football*. An irresistible quote from it, is as follows:[2]

> ... the peculiar attractiveness of football is due in some measure to the joy of rude personal encounter, face to face opposition of two hostile forces, swift flight and pursuit, tackling and dodging, kicking and catching the ball, and that the explanation of these unique pleasures must rest upon anthropological grounds. The game is more sport because the activities are more primitive. (p 31)

Gilbert, on the other hand, went on to train and practise as a psychiatrist with an interest in what nowadays would be called 'transsexual behaviour'.

Indefatigable Randy

Forward now, by 70 years, to January 1964, and San Diego, when Randy Gardner, a 17-year-old schoolboy, was determined to beat the world record of 260 hours without sleep—4 hours short of 11 days. Since his early youth he had been fascinated by 'extremes', and enjoyed the challenge of difficult projects, especially if they 'could not be done'. He was healthy, clearly self-assured and confident, and unsurprisingly described himself as 'a little on the egotistical side'. A local science fair was to be held near his home, which seemed to be a good opportunity for his marathon. Although his parents were understandably apprehensive, they were encouraging. He set his target at 264 hours, and enlisted the aid of two friends who worked shifts to keep him awake, which they succeeded in doing, because his goal was reached. It remains unbroken as the longest documented account of continuous sleep loss, although there are other, questionable claims to this. Remarkably, he took no stimulant drugs or even coffee. At first the news media knew nothing about this, but they soon became interested and increasingly encouraged him and his supporters to succeed.

On his second day he had difficulty in focusing his eyes, which became extremely heavy and tired, and thereafter he had to stop watching television for the rest of the experiment. It was not until the fourth day that more problems arose, when he became irritable and uncooperative, had memory lapses and slurred speech, and his impaired concentration became marked. He had the imaginary feeling of a tight band around his head and began to see 'fog' around street lamps. The following night he had the delusion that a street sign was a person, and shortly afterwards he thought he was a great football player, becoming resentful when people disputed this. Now five days into the study, sleep scientists got to know about him and began making medical and other tests—but there was never any real cause for concern about his health.[1]

By the sixth day, his daydreams were very evident, for example, about non-existent plants in a garden. His speech had deteriorated into to a slow, soft, slurred incoherence, and by day 9 his thoughts were fragmented and, often, he could not complete sentences. Blurred vision was a particular problem, and during the last two days he believed that people were trying to make him seem foolish because he kept forgetting things. Throughout the 11 days, the early morning hours were the most difficult when sleepiness and all the associated problems were much worse, especially very dry eyes and stuffy nose. His blood pressure and pulse remained normal, although his body temperature had fallen by an unalarming 1.0°C. A heart murmur was detected, but this was not a cause for concern and disappeared by the second recovery day. He lost all facial expression, and although this might have suggested some neurological disorder, he could, with effort, still muster up the energy to smile, which was a healthy sign. He had some hand tremor and occasional involuntary jerks in his upper arms. However, his hand co-ordination was hardly affected, and nor was his balance or walking. At no time did he show true psychotic behaviour or lose contact with reality.

The key to Randy's ability to stay awake was his determination to succeed, coupled with all the support and encouragement from those around him. Cold showers, physical activity, particularly walking, and having something interesting or exciting to do were the best ways of staying awake, which brought him back almost to normality for a while. This is best illustrated by what happened on the last night of the deprivation. He and two of his experimenters went for a walk in San Diego, from midnight to 5am, after 230 hours of deprivation, when it was noted that there was little in his behaviour to suggest that he had been awake longer than his companions. At one point, in an all-night restaurant, the three of them competed in a game on a pinball machine, with Randy holding his own in every way.

Having reached his goal he went to bed and slept for almost 15 hours, waking up spontaneously and feeling well, but somewhat sleepy. All of the difficulties that he experienced with speech, memory, daydreaming, etc, had disappeared. Over the next two nights he took an extra six and a half hours of sleep beyond his normal amount, that is, four hours extra on the second night and two and a half hours extra on the third night. Although we do not know what happened to his sleep in the ensuing days, apparently it was almost back to normal. In total he regained no more than a quarter of the sleep that he lost—an amount similar to that seen by Patrick and Gilbert and typical of more contemporary findings.

Famous four

What have these famous studies to tell us about sleep? Some say very little, because only a total of four people were involved, and what was found may be the exception rather than the rule. Possibly, but the numerous subsequent studies have found nothing remarkably different, and so let us give credit where credit is due, especially as these early findings provide us with important clues about sleep, quickly summarised thus: the real effects were confined to behaviour, with few if any physical effects and nothing of clinical significance; body temperature fell a little; the daily changes in the body clock were maintained; and, in particular, recovery was rapid following only a relatively small amount of recovery sleep in comparison with that lost. Above all, and unlike the rats in the animal studies that I described, these four participants probably enjoyed the challenge and seemed not to be particularly stressed during what must have been seen more as an adventure than as an ordeal.

The clear changes to our behaviour during sleep loss again point to our sleep having its main role within the brain, or rather the cortex, wherein our 'human' behaviour lies. In effect, progressive sleep loss turns us into automatons and, in losing the ability to think independently, conscious awareness of ourselves is impaired and we are no longer prescient. Nevertheless, we can still run on 'autopilot' and perform routine behaviour and other well-rehearsed tasks and procedures—such as the pinball game that Randy was able to play even after ten days without sleep.

Statistically significant

Since these earlier studies, most sleep deprivation experiments have been more systematic, with larger numbers of participants and greater restrictions placed upon them, largely for reasons of greater experimental precision and to ensure their safety. As a result, the situation can become more impersonal with less privacy. But by doing this, experimenters can, unwittingly, create further problems. Most studies begin with a 'baseline' condition, when the various measures are taken before the deprivation begins. Sometimes, the participants show more signs of stress than during the sleep loss itself. This rather odd finding is easily explained, because they are apprehensive about what might happen during the sleep deprivation, and worry about whether or not they will cope. Moreover, the experimenters running the experiment may also be agitated at the start, worrying about whether the equipment will work and whether their participants will stay the course. Such feelings can easily and inadvertently be transmitted to the volunteers, adding further to their worry, and raising their cortisol levels. However, after the first night of sleep loss everyone begins to relax and settle into the routine. The participants begin to see that the situation is not as bad as they may have first thought, and the experimenters become more confident—hence the subsidence of this initial stress. Several studies have certainly been affected in this way, with the investigators being perplexed as to why stress and cortisol levels fell during the first days of sleep deprivation.

Well-designed sleep loss studies should include a 'control group' of volunteers who are not sleep deprived but experience everything else. For example, both groups undergo the same baseline, normal sleep conditions without knowing whether they will be assigned to the control or to sleep deprivation conditions. They are randomly assigned to one or other of the groups, which also means that the experimenters do not know beforehand either—thus removing more potential bias. Next, both groups undergo the same measurements except that one is sleep deprived and the other is not. By comparing changes from baseline for both groups, as well as comparing between the two groups during the sleep deprivation, we can get a better idea of stress versus sleep deprivation effects. Sadly, even some recent studies have failed to take these sensible precautions.

Which finally brings me on to the often used, but often misleading, expression, 'statistically significant'. It declares whether or not a finding is important from a statistical point of view, whereby the outcome is genuine rather than just the result of chance. But it does not tell us whether the outcome is really important—if it is of medical concern, for example. Small changes can be statistically significant but of no clinical relevance, especially if they fall within the normal range of that measure for healthy individuals—and so nothing really to get excited about. To give a simple example, if a group of twenty healthy people underwent a night of sleep loss and, when compared with a control group who slept normally, they all showed a tiny fall in body temperature of 0.2°C, then statistically this would be highly significant and one could justifiably claim that sleep loss causes a significant fall in body temperature. On the face of it, this might be a cause for concern, with possibly absurd claims that sleep loss puts a severe strain on the body's ability to control its temperature. In fact, this change is trivial and of no clinical significance, and such a subsequent claim exaggerated and alarmist. Sadly, such a scenario is all too common, and we should always ask the question when hearing about findings of statistical significance, 'so what?'.

In Chapter 3 I mentioned that sleep deprivation can produce changes to aspects of our immune system that may well be statistically significant. These are not, however, necessarily good or bad, but best described as the immune system changing to suit the circumstances. Again, I emphasise that all this depends on the extent to which sleep deprivation is otherwise stressful. People who overwork and burn the candle at both ends become stressed and also lose sleep. This stress raises the body's cortisol levels, which, in turn, depresses immunity and increases the likelihood of catching colds and other infections. It is all too easy to blame all this on the lost sleep, when a stressful lifestyle may be the underlying cause of both the poor sleep and the coughs and sneezes.

There are recent experiments suggesting that even a single night of sleep loss might produce adverse effects on the heart and blood pressure, as well as producing minor diabetic-like reactions. For example, keeping people awake overnight by encouraging them to play exciting video-games, while a control group just sleeps, leads to an inevitable rise in blood pressure during the sleep loss, which can all too easily be blamed on the sleep deprivation, not on the game playing! One might then allude to the higher rate of heart disease in shift workers being caused by insufficient sleep, as has indeed been claimed. The media may pick up on such unwitting remarks from inadequate experiments, perhaps leading to unnecessary alarm. What is overlooked is that, outside the laboratory, people who in real life have poor or inadequate sleep often have troubled lives, strained relationships, other pressures, and maybe poor diets, little exercise, and being more likely to be smokers.

A recent study took patients diagnosed with high blood pressure and deprived them of sleep for a night, only to find a further, seemingly worrying rise in blood pressure, compared with a night of normal sleep. Apprehension certainly increases blood pressure, and one can only wonder about what these patients were told before the study and how any anxieties about being kept awake in hospital overnight were dealt with.

On the other hand, the many well-conducted laboratory studies of sleep deprivation might seem too artificial for any conclusions about the real effects of sleep loss to be drawn. We read claims in the press that we now live in a '24 hour 7 day' society, whereby many people are suffering from 'chronic sleep debt', and that many of the current ills might be laid at the foot of this debt. In Chapter 18, I lay out my counter-arguments to this notion. Suffice it to say that chronic sleep loss is all too easily blamed for causing serious illnesses such as heart disease, diabetes, high blood pressure, and stroke. Although sleep debt can have associations, proof that sleep deprivation is the root cause of these diseases is another matter.

Finally, another recent example of how we need to be cautious in assuming that a statistically significant effect may be of major clinical concern, comes from findings that children and adults who are shorter sleepers are liable to become obese, for whatever reason, and with the implication that short sleep poses a serious risk for obesity. For example, a large study[3] of 5–6 year old children who slept less than 10 hours a day found that they were twice as likely to be obese than those who slept more than this amount. It sounds alarming, and indeed 5.4% of these shorter sleepers were obese, compared with the 2.8% who slept for longer. On the other hand, of course, 94.6% of these shorter sleepers and 97.2% of the longer sleepers were not obese, and it would be wrong to assume that the only route to leanness is through longer sleep. The same situation applies to adults, where another large survey[4] found that 32–49 year-olds sleeping less than 7 hours a night were significantly more likely to be obese, which again suggested that more sleep might be a solution. However 77% of them were not obese, compared with 83% non-obesity for those sleeping more than 7 hours. Put this way, the differences are minor and, in fact, there are as likely to be similar proportions of obese people who are long sleepers as there are short sleepers.

Odd behaviour

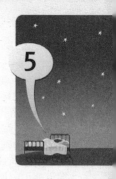

The floor seems wavy

Randy Gardner showed little sign of abnormal or psychotic behaviour, and nor did Patrick and Gilbert's participants or for that matter most other people in sleep deprivation experiments. This is an important point because it has been claimed that sleep loss produces models of madness, or 'artificial psychoses', that can be used to study psychiatric illnesses. So it has been reasoned (by others) that we could learn more about these illnesses by studying normally healthy, but sleep-deprived, people. This idea largely arose through a misunderstanding of various odd behaviours seen during sleep deprivation studies, and an unwarranted interest in the rare individual who does show apparently psychotic tendencies. In these cases it is usually discovered (too late) that the individual had some sort of psychological problem to begin with, and one might wonder why any well-balanced individual would want to volunteer for some of these arduous studies in the first place, even though they are well looked after and can pull out at any time. One sleep deprivation study actually used hospitalised patients with schizophrenia and, to the apparent surprise of the investigators, the deprivation caused a psychotic flare-up.

The best example of whom not to study under sleep loss was Peter Tripp, who, before Randy Gardner's marathon, held the record for sleep loss. He was a disc jockey, and in 1959 managed to stay awake for 201 hours while remaining in a broadcasting booth in New York's Times Square—in full public view. Given these rather bizarre circumstances, it might be expected that things might go wrong, and indeed they did. On the fourth day he was rude and abusive and started to experience waking dreams. The following day he became paranoid, thought he was being poisoned, ran off into the street, and nearly got hit by a bus. Nevertheless, with considerable help and forbearance from his supporters, he even continued to broadcast periodically and to an ever-increasing and bemused audience. Having reached his 200-hour goal, he slept almost 24 hours continuously, when he seemed quite recovered. But his friends noticed that his personality seemed to have changed for the worse. He lost his job, his wife left him, and he became a drifter. At the time, several well-known psychiatrists attributed much of what happened to him to the sleep deprivation, and used this as evidence that sleep loss causes madness. However, it turned out that Peter Tripp had a prior psychiatric history, and during the marathon he had been taking large doses of a stimulant drug related to amphetamine—known to cause personality changes.

In my own work, we have sleep deprived mentally normal and physically healthy people for up to 72 hours, and have seen outbursts of irritability or periods when participants have become withdrawn, especially in those who are rather introverted and shy, or excitable and extraverted. We now screen these individuals out, not because we worry about them, because we have never seen anything serious develop, but simply because they can be disruptive to the group and upset everybody else.

It is common for very sleepy people to have visual misperceptions, such as those reported by Patrick and Gilbert and by Randy Gardner. Such experiences are fairly trivial; nevertheless, a rating scale for rating the level of misperception was developed years ago by researchers at the Walter Reed Medical Center in Washington, renowned in the 1960s for its work into sleep loss. The scale is shown in Table 1, because it best illustrates what can happen. A score of 5 occurs only occasionally when total sleep loss usually has exceeded five days, and indicates that the person is believing what he or she has seen. We have never witnessed this in our studies. However, any unshakable belief that the misperception is real is of concern, because this belief can be psychotic like. It is mentally much healthier for one to realise that any misperceptions are just imaginations. Usually, these misperceptions and the 'tricks of the night', often seen by night sentries, are the result of the surroundings being so tediously dull, so that the

Table 1 Visual Misperception Scale for Sleep Deprivation

1 Eyes itching, burning or tired; difficulty seeing, blurred vision or diplopia

2 Visual illusions: changes in or loss of shape, size, movement, colour, or texture constancies; disturbed depth perception
   Examples:
   'The floor seems wavy'
   'The light seems to flicker'
   'The size and colour of the chairs seem to change'

3 Labelling of illusions, but with no doubt about their illusory character
   Examples:
   'Looks like fog around the light'
   'That black mark looked like it was changing into different rock formations'

4 Labelling of illusions with some doubt about their reality
   Examples:
   'I thought there was fuzz around the bottle'
   'I thought steam was rising from the floor, so I tested my eyes to check whether it was real'

5 Labelling of illusions (hallucinations) with, for a time at least, belief in their reality.
   Examples:
   'I saw hair in my milk. The others said there wasn't any but I still felt there was and would not drink it'
   'That card looked like an envelope. I turned it over to check and it had my name and address on it' (not true)

brain becomes 'fed up' with looking at the same uninteresting views and begins to liven things up a bit!

Such misperceptions can wrongly be called hallucinations, which is an overstatement, because the latter should apply only to experiences comparable to scale point 5 and worse. Even point 5 is still relatively trivial as hallucinations go. Nevertheless, because psychotic patients hallucinate, especially those with schizophrenia, mistaken links have been drawn between this disorder and these sleep deprivation effects in normal people—that is, both seem to hallucinate. Not only is there a major difference between these two types of individual in the extent of their experiences, but, more importantly, the types of hallucination that the patients have are mostly auditory, not visual, as in healthy sleep deprivation. Typically, the patients not only hear voices, but also believe in what the voices are saying to them. Few sleep deprivation studies have reported even the most minor of auditory hallucinations.

Brain washing?

Sleep-deprived volunteers are usually kept within the dull confines of a laboratory which, together with the tedium, can hasten the onset of minor visual misperceptions at levels 2 and 3, especially if the lighting is poor. So we do not really know to what extent the misperceptions are the result of the monotony, the sleep deprivation, or both. Another factor to bear in mind is that sleep deprivation can have a peculiar effect in increasing suggestibility, because a sleepy and confused state can easily lead people into believing something that they would dismiss under normal circumstances. By the way, this suggestibility is not the same as hypnotic suggestibility, and there is no evidence that sleep-deprived people are more hypnotisable.

Suggestibility during sleep deprivation is often thought to be the key to 'brain washing' in prisoners of war, but the sleep loss itself probably plays only a minor part in that wretched procedure, compared with the prolonged solitary confinement, continuous light, loss of contact with reality, depersonalisation, and severe stress. Under happier circumstances, any peculiar belief acquired during sleep loss usually disappears after a good sleep. Nevertheless, during the benign laboratory studies of sleep deprivation, experimenters may unwittingly lead their participants into thinking that certain things may happen, including experiencing misperceptions, especially by asking leading questions, such as 'Have you had any misperceptions yet?'. Not surprisingly, misperceptions will appear more readily as a result of this greater suggestibility.

The irritability that often appears during sleep deprivation studies can also be seen as a further symptom of psychosis and support for the 'artificial psychosis' idea. However, some degree of irritability is natural with sleepiness. The monotony and confinement of the experiment, with repetition of what to the participant can seem to be senseless tests, are aggravating and all too easily worsened by sleep loss. Experimenters may become flustered and socially inept with the participants, who may further argue and fall out with each other. Any irritable outburst has to be taken within the context of the actual study—a factor all too easily overlooked when reporting the outcome. Another symptom of psychosis can be suspiciousness, which is not unusual with sleep loss studies because the suspicion could be well founded, especially in those studies where the experimenter avoids telling the participants exactly what is going on, so as not to prejudice the outcome of a test!

Irritability, suspiciousness, and their knock-on effects are illustrated by the contrast between two reported studies. One (remaining nameless) involved five days without sleep, strict military-type discipline, with vigorous sports, tactical problems, night marches, etc. The other was the friendly, everybody-is-equal approach of the Walter Reed experiments mentioned earlier. Coincidentally, or otherwise, chaos broke out in the former study, with widespread irritability among participants, several unprovoked fights, gross feelings of persecution, several participants pulling out, and the study was eventually abandoned. Although none of this happened with the Walter Reed experiments, maybe the first study paints a more realistic picture of what happens during sleep loss under real-life situations, whereas the latter was too artificial and cosseted!

The largest, longest study

The longest study involving more than one person happened in September 1966, at the Neuropsychiatric Institute of the University of California at Los Angeles. Participants were to be paid quite well, and an advertisement at a student employment bureau brought forward seven volunteers, all in their early twenties. Two were rejected on health grounds and one other pulled out when he eventually understood what was involved. The remaining four, all men, were in excellent physical shape, and seemingly in good mental health, although it turned out that one 'led an extremely unstable existence' in childhood, became progressively withdrawn during the study, and needed much support from the others. Shortly after successfully completing the study, he was arrested for being a Navy deserter, which, as will be seen, was probably the most interesting outcome from the otherwise fairly uneventful study!

A large and impressive variety of measures were undertaken within a spacious, comfortable, air-conditioned, well-lit laboratory, with a TV, table tennis, and music centre. Friendly experimenters were always around. To help keep them awake, the participants had alcohol rubs, and periodically immersed their faces in bowls of ice cubes and water. They ate very well—in fact remarkably well—because at their request the daily calorie intake was double the amount needed, even taking into consideration the extra meal at night needed for being awake rather than asleep. Why this was so was not clear—it could have been through boredom, but they were kept fairly busy. I have noticed from my own experiments that sleep-deprived people do want to eat much more and I am struck by the similarities, here, with the voracious eating of the sleep-deprived rats at the Chicago Sleep Laboratory. But given that these humans remained quite healthy, such similarities may simply be a coincidence. A more likely reason may be through the hormonal link between feeding and sleeping discussed in Chapter 3.

Anyway, to return to this particular study, the volunteers had to go without sleep for nine days (eight nights), which they all accomplished. Even then, at the end of their endurance, all thought that a further 24 hours could still be just possible—if they were paid enough! The offer was declined by the experimenters, who were themselves worn out. For the participants, debilitating sleepiness did not set in until the third day, when, for example, reading became impossible. By the fourth day irritability was common; by the fifth day conversation and social interaction had largely ceased, and misperceptions were at their worst. The only instance of what might be seen as a true visual hallucination was when one of them temporarily went 'berserk' during a tedious task of tracking a spot of light across a screen. He suddenly screamed in terror and fell to the floor sobbing and muttering incoherently about a gorilla. He had begun to fall asleep during the task, with what seems to have been a sudden onset of rapid eye movement (REM) sleep and an accompanying nightmare. The investigators were obviously very concerned and one, a psychiatrist, interviewed him when he had gathered his senses shortly afterwards. He confessed to having a similar experience in his sleep when a child, with the recurrent theme of Humpty Dumpty being attacked by a gorilla. When he was staring at that spot of light the scene changed in this manner, which had already happened several times during the experiment, but he had felt too embarrassed to mention it. Having talked about the problem, he was able to return to the task and, after another similar episode, it seemed to disappear.

Euphoria

Many mentally healthy people become quite euphoric during the first night of sleep deprivation and get quite a 'buzz' from it, especially if they are having a late night party (even without the alcohol!). However, there is usually no enduring effect after having some recovery sleep. Interestingly, a night of total or partial sleep loss (for example, only four hours of sleep) can be beneficial to those people suffering from very severe forms of depression.[1] Rapid mood improvement occurs in about two-thirds of these sufferers and, in some, the effects are dramatic, with patients becoming quite euphoric to the extent that this type of sleep deprivation has been used as a therapy, usually in conjunction with antidepressant medication. Unfortunately, these remarkable improvements usually disappear quickly with ensuing sleep, sometimes even following a short nap. Nevertheless, patients find the experience helpful because they realise that, despite what may be months or years of suffering from this debilitating disorder, their normal behaviour is still there, somewhere, and intact in the recesses of their minds. Better still, they see that there is still the possibility that their normal behaviour will be retrieved quite quickly. I must emphasise that these mood-improving effects are apparent only during the sleep loss and, unfortunately, the increasing sleepiness brings on the struggle to remain awake, and the rather different misery that this brings with it. But the improved mood at the time more than compensates. Patients responding best to this form of treatment are those who usually show some improvement in mood over the day, as well as those with a marked variation in their depression from day to day.

As a result of this accompanying sleepiness, depressed patients undergoing this sleep deprivation 'therapy' have to be supervised for their safety, and for this reason the treatment is not very practical, especially with outpatients. Also, it pays to be cautious about the extent to which the sleep loss itself improves depression. There is a real effect of some sort, but the problem with these studies is that, in order to keep the patients awake, the medical staff have to interact with them to a much greater extent than usual—which may well be another reason why the patients become more cheerful. The problem with this research is that it is difficult to control for this latter effect. What would be interesting is for the medical staff to interact much more with these same patients during a normal day, without sleep loss. Regrettably, such procedures are usually too costly in terms of staff and their time.

Paradoxically, one of the symptoms of depression is waking up early in the morning. Given the potential benefits of sleep deprivation, it suggests that this early awakening ought to be therapeutic. But it is not, although it has been suggested that if it was not for the early morning awakening the depression would be worse, and that early awakening is 'nature's' attempt to limit the depression. This nice idea lacks solid evidence in its support and, besides, the early morning wakening usually still allows for five or six hours of sleep, which is probably too much to be of any benefit to the depression.

The opposite extreme to severe depression is mania. During periods of mania, which can last for several weeks, sufferers tend to sleep very little, and what is even more interesting is that they do not seem to be very sleepy. This again points to a fascinating link between mood and sleep length, but exactly what is happening in the brain, to explain this, is little understood. For example, prescribing sleeping tablets to lengthen sleep is not a treatment for mania. In Chapter 17, I come back to this topic, because mentally healthy, natural short sleepers can also have a mild form of 'exuberance', which they can turn to their advantage.

Skin and bones

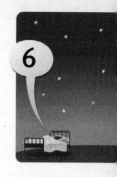

Do we grow in our sleep?

Well, yes and no. Measure your height before going to sleep and again immediately on awakening next morning and there is an extra centimetre or more. Unfortunately, soon after getting up and walking around, it has gone! Lying down for several hours, whether it be asleep or awake, allows the cartilaginous discs between the vertebrae to absorb water, expand a little, and lengthen the backbone. Standing up afterwards causes the body's weight and gravity to compress the discs once more. This applies particularly to children, and even to the length of their arms and legs, because physical rest allows the more 'spongy' cartilaginous ends of the limb bones, where the growth occurs, to absorb water and lengthen a little. However, the activity of wakefulness again squeezes this water out.

The sequence of events in a child's body that cause it to grow remain unclear. There is evidence that growth spurts are accompanied by more sleep, but we do not know which is causing what, and it is possible that some other factor is causing both to happen. Having said this, I should mention that a hormone intimately involved with growth, not surprisingly called 'growth hormone', is produced in relatively large quantities in the early part of normal sleep in both the child and the adult. The hormone certainly helps growth in children but not really in the adult. Staying awake, when the hormone usually reaches its peak, will suppress it, but other, smaller surges will now appear during wakefulness. Given this hormone's name, one could easily deduce that growth and repair are indeed stimulated by sleep. But this sleep-related hormone surge is rare in other mammals, even for those with similar sleep patterns to ours, such as the dog and cat.

Other hormones intimately involved with the growth process, such as insulin, are not so dependent on sleep.

The most rapid growth spurt, in adolescence, is also when daily sleep usually becomes markedly longer. However tempting it may be to make a direct connection, there is as yet no hard evidence for this and no indication that this particular growth spurt is confined to sleep. Coupled with the adolescent's predilection for going to bed later, the factor most associated with their sleep is not so much growth but more mundane matters of the all too-familiar problems of getting the grumpy teenager up for morning school.

Beauty and radiance

But what about beauty sleep and those wrinkles that are supposed to vanish with sleep overnight? Indeed, they may disappear, because sleep (rather than just lying down) causes the face and forehead to perspire more than usual, with more water being retained within the skin to puff it up and flatten those wrinkles. Alas, morning arising and greater exposure to the air dry the skin out and the wrinkles pop back. Many so-called anti-wrinkle creams applied at night simply allow the skin to retain more of this water and help keep it puffed up for longer in the morning, but do not actually remove or prevent wrinkles. By the way, the skin just below the eyes is particularly thin and more vulnerable to being puffed up like this during sleep, causing some people to wake up with noticeable bags under their eyes, which soon flatten out next morning. The problem is that all this stretching and contraction of the skin will eventually produce all too many wrinkles under the eyes.

When we sleep, and even when we are awake, it is usually the face that is most exposed to the air, and because of this we can lose a surprisingly large amount of heat from our faces. That is why, when we become hot and need to cool down, the cheeks and forehead easily become red, because the skin here contains a rich supply of tiny blood vessels (capillaries) that expand with warm blood—hence the flushing. Heat from the blood in the cheeks radiates through the thin layer of skin above and is lost to the outside. Even more heat can be lost through perspiration or, rather, from the evaporation of the perspired water (called 'latent heat loss'), especially from the cheeks and forehead. The body continually produces heat during sleep, as it does in wakefulness, and to stop overheating it has to lose excess heat, which it can do fairly effectively from the exposed face, because the rest of the body is usually too well insulated by clothes or bedding.

Blood moves heat around the body (just like hot water in central heating and car cooling systems) and dumps it through its cheek radiators. Losing heat just before sleep is important because the body likes to cool down a little (by about 0.3°C) then, as this helps the process of falling asleep. It is the reason why our cheeks are often flushed at bedtime. To be more precise, it is the brain that likes to be cooler at this time, and facial flushing is particularly good at doing this through a rather amazing process—the cooled blood from the flushed cheeks drains into a special vein, which can just be seen as that blue patch close to the skin surface in the inside corners of each eye. From there it goes into the large jugular veins of the neck, returning this and other blood from the head, back to the heart. The trick is that the jugulars, containing their cooler blood, lie alongside the main (carotid) arteries, sending warm blood up to the brain from deep within the body. Whereas it is a bad idea to have your domestic cold water pipe running alongside the hot water one, as heat is lost from the hot to the cold pipe, it is a good idea for the blood entering the brain from the carotids to be cooled by being so close to the jugular veins in this 'counter-current cooling system'! There is more to be said for keeping a cool head for sleep, and I pick up this topic again when I come to insomnia in Chapter 20, because we can exploit it to improve sleep.

Although the rest of the body perspires during sleep (to a lesser extent than the face), this moisture just gets absorbed by the bedclothes. Interestingly, we seem to perspire quite a lot when asleep, even under cool bedroom conditions. Perspiration is largely under the control of the brain, which puts some restriction on perspiration when we are awake. However, for some unknown reason, during sleep this restriction is lifted and body perspiration increases, which is why we may easily lose half a litre or more of perspiration during the course of the night. All this water does not go to waste, however, because it is enjoyed by the teeming numbers of minute fungi and mites that invariably occupy your bed and mattress, which feast on the millions of sloughed off, dead skin cells. These unwanted guests do appreciate a drink with their meal!

Night starvation

Keeping to the topic of food, many people believe that the body needs to stock up on supplies to keep it going through the small hours in order to stave off 'night starvation'. One reason for this is the belief that sleep aids general body recovery after the wear and tear of wakefulness—a notion largely based on the misinterpretation of various bodily events in sleep. As we have seen, sleep, rather than relaxed wakefulness, is essential to the cortex, but any special benefit that sleep has for the rest of the body is another matter. Remember, Randy Gardner showed no physical ill-effects or lack of 'body repair' during sleep deprivation, and nor has anyone else who is only sleep deprived and not otherwise stressed.

As mammals go, adult human sleep is unusual, because it is rather lengthy and because our last meal of the day is usually early evening, with much of it digested by the early hours. If we were not asleep then, we would be hungry and want to eat—which is exactly what happens with the night-shift worker. Similarly, the person with insomnia will often feel quite peckish at this time and in need of some sustenance—so why do we not naturally wake up in the middle of the night to eat?

One response might be that being awake uses up more energy, hence the increased need to eat. But this is not the answer, because simply sitting around, using up little more energy than being asleep, also brings on this hunger. The sleeping body has a contingency plan to avoid waking in the middle of the night, because the feeling of hunger is suppressed by sleep and, as an alternative to eating, the body releases and utilises some of its stored energy reserves, especially in body fat. Above, I mentioned growth hormone, and here is where it seems to play its key role. Before explaining further I should mention that few other mammals fast in their sleep as we do. For example, cows, sheep, and other herbivores continue to ruminate and digest their food throughout sleep, carnivores gorge themselves on meat, which can take up to a day to digest, and rodents wake up periodically to nibble more food. Whereas we show a large surge in growth hormone during our sleep, these other animals do not have this, probably because there is always digested food available. Our unique growth hormone surge in sleep prevents night starvation by causing metabolism to turn to our reserves of body fat and utilise this to 'stoke the body fire'—in one sense we can slim by sleeping! Staying awake instead prevents this hormone surge; the fat remains intact and hence the need for that night-time feed. So, we do not have to eat heartily at bedtime, and those milky drinks should be seen as a pleasure and maybe a comforter in the case of children, but not as a necessity to ward off night-time hunger or starvation.

'Breakfast' (a shortening of 'breaking fast') is aptly named, and probably why the English indulge in a large breakfast, or at least they used to. At the other end of the day, as was once common across Europe, one did not take one's supper (from the Latin *suppare*, for soup) until late at night, after having had one or two hours' sleep in the early evening. Supper was seen to be the most important meal of the day with family and friends gathered together. Falling asleep, then, was most impolite to say the least, because it was essential to be alert and have good conversation with one's fellow diners. A sleep beforehand ensured that one was on top form and able to stay up late. The ensuing night's (somewhat shortened) sleep, on a full stomach, meant that one could still rise with the dawn, feeling refreshed and only needing a small meal—as implied by the French term for breakfast—'le petit déjeuner'—more about mediaeval sleeping habits in Chapter 18.

Renewal

When most of the billions of cells in our bodies grow to a certain size they usually divide into two; this is not an automatic process, however, because it can be delayed for one reason or another. Although cells usually divide throughout the 24-hour day, this process is influenced by the body's 24-hour clock, with a typical peak of cell division being at around 2am. Feeding also leads to a rise in cell division several hours afterwards, when the food has been digested and the nutrients absorbed into the bloodstream, to be taken up by these cells for their growth. This 2am peak coincides not only with sleep but also with the surge in growth hormone mentioned above. Putting two and two together to make five, and given this hormone's name, it might be assumed that the daily peak in cell division is caused by sleep. The problem with this idea is that, if one stays awake at 2am, but rests instead of sleeping (which means that there is no increase in growth hormone, because it is sleep related), the peak in cell division remains. That is because cell division requires physical rest (not necessarily sleep), and is largely governed by both our 24-hour clock and prior food intake—no food and this peak is diminished.

I should mention that there is also another, smaller peak in cell division, some hours after lunch, mid-afternoon, and largely as a result of lunch. It is more apparent when we sit relaxed, awake, but we do not have to be asleep, despite our propensity for a mid-afternoon nap. Afternoon sleepiness is not caused by lunch and is still present when lunch is missed, although, if lunch is particularly heavy and taken with something alcoholic, a nap is almost inevitable!

Whereas physical rest permits cell division, exercise slows it up—which is why, in rodents, their daily peak in cell division is constrained to their sleep. Again, it is not sleep itself that causes this peak, but the physical inactivity of sleep. Remember, these animals have little relaxed wakefulness and are always on the go, unless they are asleep. Hence, their peaks in cell division are delayed until the inactivity of sleep. I should not really compare children with rodents, although some parents might like to do so at times. Nevertheless, in that children also tend to be very active in wakefulness, it is likely that much of their cell division is also delayed until sleep, for the same reason as for the rodent.

Cells die. Some types of cells live only for days (such as red blood cells), most for months, whereas others, such as brain and heart cells, usually last throughout one's lifetime. Given that body tissues and organs are made of cells, physical growth of these tissues—let us say bone and skin—must entail more cells being produced (by cell division) than being lost by dying. It can be likened to the population of a country, because the birth rate (akin to cell division) does not tell you how many people exist—this also depends on how many have died at that time. A rapid rise in the birth rate does not necessarily mean that the population is growing, because more deaths than births means that total numbers are declining. My point is, returning to sleep, that cell death rates are not particularly linked to sleep or wakefulness, but rather to the body clock. The net effect is that we do not seem to have more body cells after sleeping or, in this respect, nor have we grown more in our sleep. Although growth spurts in children are linked to 'sleep spurts', as I mentioned at the beginning of this chapter, the growth spurts are probably not caused by sleep.

7 Sleepiness

Feeding the mind

In Chapter 1, I mentioned that the cortex is unable to switch off and rest to any marked extent, outside sleep. On the other hand, many brain structures below the cortex, largely controlling vital body functions and common to all mammals, continue to function fairly normally throughout sleep, as in wakefulness. Unlike the cortex, most if not all of these areas seem neither to sleep nor to need it, even though they may influence sleep in one way or another. They tell us little about the purpose of sleep—but rather, how it is regulated.

We have all been without sleep on some occasion and know what it is like—just as Gilbert experienced it over 100 years ago. To view sleepiness simply as a lack of sleep seems reasonable, but it is as helpful as saying that the function of sleep is simply to eliminate sleepiness, or that, because coffee with its caffeine can overcome sleepiness, at least for a while, caffeine must be as good as sleep. To demonstrate how much more there is to sleepiness, let me illustrate this with hunger, which is similar to sleepiness in many ways. Go without food and we get hungry; eat and hunger goes. So we eat just to eliminate hunger, which again seems a reasonable notion, but it is only a superficial view. What exactly is hunger? It comprises stomach pangs, sensations of hunger, increasing thoughts about eating, looking for food, and, eventually, physical weakness. However, there is mind over matter here, because both hunger and searching for food will disappear without eating, at least for a while, if we are distracted by something else of greater interest.

Let me continue with the hunger analogy. We can measure it in various ways. For example, monitor the stomach's pangs by placing sensors on the skin over the abdomen. This is an 'objective' method, because our thoughts should not, in theory at least, be able to influence these pangs (although they do!). In contrast, a truly 'subjective' method would be to ask the person to rate their feelings of hunger on a scale, such as:

1=definitely not hungry
2=not hungry
3=not sure
4=a bit hungry
5=hungry
6=very hungry, cannot think of anything else.

But are they being honest? We could be more subtle and have an 'eating latency test', by putting people in a room with a table of attractive foods and see how long it takes them to start eating. Then record how much they eat—the theory being that the greater the hunger the sooner they start eating and the more they eat. Of course, our participants might be very hungry, but restrain themselves for one reason or another—perhaps not wanting to appear impolite or greedy. On the other hand, they may not be hungry at all, but rush to the table because they are greedy!

Unfortunately, none of these measures tells us what the purpose of hunger really is. To do so we would have to wait until something else happened following prolonged hunger, which would be weakness, and then we could delve into what caused it. For example, take blood samples and look at blood sugar and hormone levels. Although these would not provide the definitive answer as to why we eat, they would certainly provide important clues.

Sleepiness can be measured by attaching sensors ('electrodes') to the scalp and monitoring the brain's electrical activity ('brainwaves') from underneath—which shows clear changes with sleepiness; this is described later. Even then, with this seemingly very scientific and objective measure, the sleepy person can exercise 'mind over matter', and decide to become more alert by thinking about something exciting, when the brainwaves will change towards alertness. An even more objective approach, perhaps, would be to put the individual in one of the sophisticated types of 'brain scanner' and take a three-dimensional picture of the workings inside the sleepy brain, to see what has changed when compared with an alert brain. Although these pictures might seem to be the ultimate in objective measurement, they remain difficult to interpret because we do not know whether the changes that are seen are the actual cause of sleepiness or just another reflection of it. It is like looking inside a mechanical clock to see why it keeps stopping—you do not know which bit is the actual cause unless you dismantle the clock in an orderly and knowledgeable way. Unfortunately, these brain imaging techniques are not yet sophisticated enough to dismantle the brain's bits safely and discover which is causing what.

A 'sleep latency test' is seen to be particularly good at measuring sleepiness, with the idea being that the more sleepy we are the quicker we will fall asleep. For this test the sleepy individual lies on a bed in a quiet and comfortable room and is asked to relax and try to go to sleep. Brainwaves are measured, as before, to detect the first signs of sleep. Although this might be an objective test, it is not foolproof, because a sleepy person might simply decide not to go to sleep or, as before, start thinking about something that worries or excites him or her, and seem more alert than is the case. I come back to this test later, in Chapter 18.

Subjectively, and at what may seem to be the 'sloppy end' of sleepiness measurement, we can ask the sleepy individual to rate his or her sleepiness on a rating scale that, again, depends on the honesty of the person concerned. Here is a well-known scale:[1]

1 = extremely alert
2 = very alert
3 = alert
4 = rather alert
5 = neither alert nor sleepy
6 = some signs of sleepiness
7 = sleepy, no effort to stay awake
8 = sleepy, some effort to stay awake
9 = very sleepy, great effort to keep awake, fighting sleep.

Of course, these descriptions also depend on whether one understands English, because translations can produce biases, whereby whole populations can seem more sleepy or alert than others.

In fact, all these measures and others that I describe have their various problems and, more to the point, even the apparently more scientific and objective approaches are not foolproof—they are either still influenced by individual whim or provide data that is, at the very least, difficult to interpret.

Spare capacity

With hunger and eating we can cope with missing a meal or two, because the body can utilise its energy stores, despite the feelings of hunger. The cortex also seems to have some capacity to cope with sleep loss despite feelings of sleepiness. Apart from using willpower to stay awake, it seems that parts of the cortex particularly affected by sleep loss can, for a while, recruit the assistance of other areas not so badly affected. An analogy comes from those advanced computers having what is known as an 'error correct' facility, whereby spare circuits are built into complex networks that can automatically be switched on if one of the usual circuits fails. The computer re-routes through the spare circuits to bypass the problem, and the computer operator notices nothing wrong because the whole system still functions normally. Failures can continue to build up, unnoticed, until the spare circuitry runs out, and only then will the operator detect a fault. At first glance this may seem to be a single, perhaps minor, problem because it is only the last fault that is apparent, but, when the system is examined in detail, not one fault is discovered, but many, and a major repair of many circuits is required.

Something similar might happen to the cortex. It must develop faults in its networks during wakefulness—after all, it is one of the most complex machines in existence. These must be bypassed somehow, during wakefulness, presumably by re-routing through other neural networks. Probably, most if not all these faults are repaired 'off line' during sleep. Now, it is reasonable to assume that there are enough spare circuits to keep us going beyond the 16 hours of one waking day, and there must be provision for a reserve capacity, especially because, when we apply more compensatory effort to the task at hand, this can usually offset the effects of sleep loss for about 30 hours of continuous wakefulness, when, despite one's best efforts, mental performance really begins to fail. Increasing this mental effort may also help switch on those spare circuits and may be a reason why interesting and stimulating tasks can withstand some sleep loss, whereas performance at simple and dull tasks results in more rapid deterioration—we cannot be bothered to apply more effort and connect up those extra circuits. There is recent evidence[2] to support this idea that cortical regions normally not involved with the task at hand can be recruited to 'help out' those regions that are failing because of prolonged wakefulness.

Microsleeps

Sleepiness has a distinct circadian rhythm, when we are at our daily worst around 4–6am, with another dip in the early afternoon. The latter is probably because we are designed to have two sleeps a day— the main one at night and a nap or longer siesta in the afternoon (see Chapter 10). In contrast there are the ups, with the high spot being around early evening when the body clock perks us up to a remarkable degree. There also tends to be a smaller surge around mid-morning. These ups and downs become more apparent with sleep loss, which prompted a famous psychologist, 50 years ago, to declare that the effects of going without sleep are 'not like a mechanical toy which goes slower as it runs down. Nor is it like a car engine which continues normally until its fuel is exhausted and then stops dead. It is like a motor which after much use misfires, runs normally for a while, then falters again' (p 2).[3]

The sleepy cortex cannot cope with monotony and becomes easily bored. To keep awake it needs stimulation, otherwise we nod off. Which is not a very profound statement, because you all know this anyway. Nevertheless, similar but rather more convoluted 'behavioural' theories about sleep were common in the nineteenth century, particularly that sleep was simply the result of an absence of external stimulation, with wakefulness being possible only if the organism was constantly stimulated. Take the stimulation away and the person or animal will fall asleep. At the turn of the twentieth century, another variation on this theme, proposed by the Frenchman, Dr Eduard Claparede, became very popular. He considered that sleep was not so much a passive response, but an active process similar to an instinct, to avoid the onset of fatigue—'we sleep not because we are intoxicated or exhausted, but in order to prevent our becoming intoxicated or exhausted' (p 427).[4] For him, sleep begins simply when we have had enough of being awake, which was an interesting idea at the time, perhaps—but that is enough of history and so let us get back to the present.

It is not surprising that the most sensitive tests of sleepiness are those that are simple, dull, and monotonous, and why so many sleep researchers focus on these tasks, with the most popular being 'simple reaction time'. This was first used by Patrick and Gilbert, as described in Chapter 4. Nowadays, more elaborate versions are used, where a light signal flashes or a 'beep' will sound, requiring an immediate response by pushing a button. The interval is the 'reaction time', and the process is repeated every 5–12 seconds (the interval has to be varied to make it less predictable), and the whole test usually lasts at least 10 minutes. It is very boring, especially when performed in a small featureless room with no distractions. Ten minutes or so of this and even the mildly sleepy person will succumb to lapses of attention. It is easy to visualise what happens here—the eyelids droop, then close, only to open again after a few seconds. This is a typical 'microsleep', when any visual stimulus from the reaction time device is missed, of course, and even a 'beep' sound may go unnoticed.

Lapses can also simply be caused by the sleepy individual desperately looking around the featureless room for some form of stimulation, only to miss a stimulus. Between these lapses or microsleeps the reaction time is almost (but not quite) back to normal. If all these individual responses are averaged together, it might seem that there is a marked slowing of all response, when in fact most of the responses are almost normal, whereas the others, the lapses, comprise a very long or nil reaction. Microsleeps seem harmless enough in these laboratory settings, but can be deadly if one happens to be driving on dull and monotonous roads, such as motorways, where about 25 per cent of all crashes are sleep related—more about driver sleepiness and lapses, later.

Reaction time tests really measure tolerance to boredom, and some might argue that they almost create the sleepiness in the first place. Although the tests are supposed to be 'objective', not easily affected by one's state of mind, this is not the case if sleepy people are given an incentive to do well, for example, by creating some sort of competition over the test. Then, participants will perk up and the lapses will diminish, or even disappear, as the task is now not so boring. All this might seem rather academic, but it is not, and here is an example of why, from the Second World War, many allied aircraft crashed on homeward flights, after bombing raids or 'dog fights'. These crashes were not always because of damage to the plane, but linked to the crew having woefully insufficient sleep before they set out, because they were constantly called into action. Whereas the 'adrenaline rush' and stimulation of the mission kept even the sleepiest flyer awake on the outward journey, when homeward bound, after the stress and excitement was over, relaxation set in and so did sleep. Despite the best efforts of these fliers to stay awake many would succumb. Even their knowing full well the danger of falling asleep and the need for willpower to stay awake, they were so sleep deprived that they could not manage to do this. Intense sensory stimulation would have helped, but none was available.

I should also add that there is no support for the idea that the more one experiences sleep deprivation the more 'immune' or tolerant one becomes. If anything, repeated sleep loss under the same circumstances becomes even more tedious and thus more difficult to withstand.

Many psychological tests are sensitive to sleepiness, such as 'working memory' tasks, whereby, for example, short strings of simple words or numbers have to be remembered and recalled soon afterwards. Another example is 'tracking' tasks, requiring the monotonous following, with a joystick, of a moving target on a screen. When we're fully alert, performance at these tests usually improves with practice, or we discover a 'knack for beating the system'. Consequently, they have to be well rehearsed beforehand, so that these effects have levelled off. Only then should the tests be used for actual sleepiness measurement, otherwise the improvement with practice, or whatever, will balance out any deterioration caused by sleepiness, leading to no net change when, in fact, sleep loss does cause a decline. Of course, 'practice makes perfect' also makes the task even more tedious when it comes to the real testing period. What is not always clear is whether these tests are sensitive to sleepiness simply because of their simplicity, monotony, and lack of inherent interest, or whether they are tapping into something more fundamental to sleep loss. The greater the unremitting tedium and apparent futility of a test, the shorter the period needed before the deterioration caused by sleepiness sets in, and for this reason some psychologists pride themselves in devising the most excruciatingly boring tasks!

In their defence, however, these tasks are of great value to sleep research because they are so sensitive to sleepiness, and much credit for their development must go to the late Dr Bob Wilkinson, who worked in Cambridge, UK, and currently to Dr David Dinges and his colleagues,[5] at the University of Pennsylvania, who have developed the very widely used 'psychomotor vigilance test' (PVT).

Demanding tasks

To explore this last point further—that sleep loss and the resultant sleepiness simply affect the ability to withstand boredom—we can give tasks that are intellectually much more exciting and interesting. If these are not affected by sleepiness, even when given for half an hour or so, it might seem that the boredom theory may be right. On the other hand, the extra effort we apply to combat the sleepiness when doing these interesting tests may pull in the spare capacity I just mentioned, which we do not bother to use for the boring tests. The third alternative, and more food for thought, is that, if some sort of very demanding task for the cerebral cortex was not affected by sleepiness, at least for a night or so of nil sleep, then maybe sleep is not of such benefit to the cortex as we have supposed. Maybe sleepiness is simply some primitive mechanism to induce sleep and keep us out of harm's way at night. If so, maybe we should look for a new, as yet unknown, sophisticated drug that might more effectively remove sleepiness, without harmful effects. Remember, the 'cruder' drugs such as amphetamines and caffeine do not remove the need for sleep, but largely mask the feeling of sleepiness—in the same way that aspirin works on a fever, by removing the symptoms but not the underlying cause.

I do not really know the answer to these alternatives. Certainly, IQ tests and other demanding tests of deductive, critical thinking are not affected by 36 hours without sleep, even when the task lasts well beyond half an hour. These tests generate much interest for the sleepy individual, but as to why they are insensitive to sleep loss remains to be seen. Part of the problem is that, because of the apparent insensitivity of these tests to sleep loss, sleep researchers have turned their backs on them and have not really pursued this line of enquiry.

Whereas demanding and motivating conditions will help overcome the effects of sleep loss, with many complex and interesting tasks being unaffected, it might be thought that this tenet also applies to all tasks, including 'high level decision-making' and innovative, flexible thinking—collectively called 'executive thinking' (nothing to do with people working as executives, by the way). This executive thinking is not the same as logical and deductive thinking, where the answer can be found through a methodical working out, but rather it is when you have to think 'outside the box' or 'think by the seat of one's pants'. To get to the point, executive thinking is indeed impaired by sleep loss, despite one's best efforts to overcome this deterioration and do well—more on this fascinating topic in Chapter 8.

The eyes have it

One does not need to be a sleep researcher to know when someone is sleepy—just look at the face, especially the eyes. Some years ago, when I was running 3-day (72-hour) total sleep deprivation studies on young adults, we took full face 'mug shots' of each participant, every 12 hours, as well as before and after deprivation. Afterwards, and for each person, the photos were shuffled up and we asked various naïve people to rate the photos in the order of increasing sleepiness. It turned out that most of these raters were very good at doing this, except when it came to rating the few participants who coped very well at all our tests during the entire deprivation, and who never looked particularly sleepy. There are inexplicable differences between people in the effects of sleep loss. Being male or female, young or old, fit or unfit, thin or plump, tall or short does not seem to provide the answer—which probably lies within the brain—and it is not simply a matter of differences in 'willpower'.

The usual key signs of worsening sleepiness are losses of facial expression and 'sadder' 'sunken' eyes with less 'sparkle'. Sleepiness slows up eye blinking, which can cause the eyes to dry out and become itchy and red. To avoid this during our sleep loss studies, we keep the room temperature pleasant but cool, and ensure that the air is relatively humid. None of our volunteers smokes, because, apart from anything else, cigarette smoke further irritates the eyes of sleepy people. As a result of all this, none of our volunteers experiences red eyes.

Yawning gaps

There are other apparent signs of sleepiness that can be quite deceptive, even to the trained observer, with the best example being yawning. Despite it being a universal human behaviour, no one really knows much about it, other than that it usually has something to do with boredom or sleepiness. Yawning can be seen in many zoo mammals, as well as in dogs, horses, and mice, for example, when it is usually accompanied by stretching. The ostrich also seems to do a lot of it, especially when drowsily sitting on its eggs.

Look up the word in a dictionary, and apart from learning that it comes from the old English verb '*ganien*'—to gape, there usually follows only bland statements of the obvious. Medical textbooks are little better, and often the subject is conspicuous by its absence—it should lie somewhere between 'yaba virus' and 'yaws'. Astute physicians and scientists lost for an explanation for a phenomenon will often give it an impressive new name, usually derived from Latin. Thus the term once commonly adopted for yawning was 'oscitation' from '*oscitare*' (to open the mouth wide), and this can be found in older medical texts. It implies that science and medicine knew all about it, and one ponderous explanation, providing an effective smoke screen to conceal ignorance is along the lines of 'a deep inspiration carried out with widely opened glottis, typically with open mouth, and frequently accompanied by movements of the arms, etc. It is caused by certain psychic influences.'

Another account comes from a medical textbook by Dr H. Russel, from New York, dated 1891, who proposed that yawning was produced by 'bad air in the lungs designed by Nature as a gymnastic to awaken the respiratory organs into activity'.[6] Similar views prevail today—that somehow yawning 'aerates' the lungs and increases the oxygen supply to the brain. However, more enlightened research has clearly shown that yawning has little to do with 'oxygenating the blood', because breathing oxygen does not suppress the urge to yawn and, conversely, raising carbon dioxide levels in the blood does not increase yawning. If anything, yawning leads not to a rise in blood oxygen levels, but a fall, because breathing usually ceases for a while after a yawn. It is also caused by stress and fear, which may account for its association with injury and severe bleeding. In the First World War, yawning was commonly seen among troops in the trenches waiting for the whistle to blow, for going 'over the top'. Heroin addicts withdrawing from the drug and going 'cold turkey', which can be a frightening experience, can yawn extensively—so can migraine sufferers before an impending migraine, which may or may not be linked to fear of the migraine attack.

The Victorians had other various theories about yawning, many of which can best be described as 'imaginative'. For example, yawning stimulates arousal by boosting blood levels of the hormone thyroxine (which raises metabolism). The yawning of the lower jaw was supposed to squeeze the thyroid gland, which is located in the neck, to release more of this hormone into the bloodstream. Certainly, yawning can cause a momentary increase in heart rate, but this is a reflex associated with any deep inspiration and is followed by a slowing on expiration.

The peak of research into yawning was in the 1920s. Notable was a Dr Carl Mayer who devoted much time to precisely measuring yawning, including taking radiographs of his wretched subjects attempting to yawn, as well as having their throats probed by laryngeal mirrors and their necks palpated. He was at pains to note that his measurements did not interfere with yawning, and declared, 'the complete yawning complex, unmodified by inhibition, was allowed to develop'. He confidently claimed that yawning could be divided into three precisely timed and distinct phases: 'initial inspiration', taking between 1.9 and 4.3 seconds, 'acme', lasting exactly 2.3 seconds, and 'expiration' of 4.5–7.8 seconds' duration. As to why we yawn, he dismissed it with two words—'cerebral fatigue'.[7]

Despite common knowledge that yawning has 'something psychological about it', surprisingly few psychologists have investigated it. Many psychiatrists have taken a keen interest, however, but often with some strange concepts. For example, in patients with schizophrenia, yawning has been taken as a sign of a good prognosis, supposedly showing that the patient wants to maintain contact with the real world. Some antidepressant medicines can produce frequent yawning, not because of increased sleepiness, but through direct effects on yawning control mechanisms in the brain.

One of the most endearing accounts of yawning was based on a series of experiments performed in 1941, by Dr Joseph Moore from the George Peabody College, in Tennessee. His first study employed a stooge, who was able to yawn at will and sat in a nearby public library reading room, in full view of other readers. He yawned obtrusively every ten minutes while Moore sat unobtrusively in an overlooking gallery, recording the events in his notebook. Within a minute or so of each rendition almost half of the unwitting audience would follow suit. Another of Moore's studies was more blatant, with a short movie of a girl yawning, shown to an unsuspecting audience, which was soon followed by a doubling of the incidence of yawning among the onlookers. His last study was more imaginative: can yawning be stimulated simply by hearing it rather than by seeing the yawner? Gramophone records of yawning were played to college students, with little response, but when played to blind students yawning became most apparent. Indeed, yawning is highly suggestible—try it now!

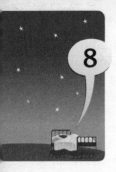

8 Higher matters

Executives

One problem with laboratory tests of sleepiness is that their relationship to real-world activities is not always evident. A good illustration concerns junior hospital doctors (interns) who suffer sleep loss and long working hours on a routine basis. Although there has been much research into the effects of sleepiness on these staff, it has tended to focus on simple tasks such as reaction time, which seem to have little to do with the true nature of their jobs. Sometimes the overall picture can be confusing, with no apparent decline in clinical skills, but with impaired reaction time and deterioration in other psychological performance tasks that are of unknown relevance to medical practice. For example, after a night of being on call, anaesthetists usually have no difficulty in monitoring 'vital signs' during an operation, although they have been found to be impaired on a psychological reasoning test. Moreover, many of these studies have been badly designed—for example, with sleep loss findings compared with off-duty days, when the clinician is still recovering from the effects of long work hours and performance is still impaired. Here, the results of sleep deprivation are underestimated because the so-called recovery days are just as bad and give little insight into performance during a medical emergency. Probably the only consistent finding has been that sleep loss affects the clinician's mood, which understandably worsens, usually with increasing irritability.

Few studies have assessed the real abilities of the sleepy doctor. One found that sleep-deprived junior doctors were more hesitant and showed less planning during a surgical procedure. Another found that anaesthetists who had minimal sleep during a night on call were less innovative in dealing with their patients, and had poorer communication skills. However, the most recent and substantial finding, coming from the USA,[1] found an almost sixfold increase in diagnostic errors made by interns while they worked extended (24 hours or more) shifts, compared with when they had more adequate sleep.

At my laboratory, we have tried to simulate real-life settings. For example, in one sleep loss study we used a competitive marketing game called 'Masterplanner'. Its aim is to promote sales for an imaginary, newly developed product—ultimately to achieve market dominance and a substantive profit in the face of increasing competition from market rivals (the competing players). Success comes with the continuing ability to handle and react to quickly changing situations, and the game particularly taps into being able to think flexibly, to be innovative, and to update plans in the light of changing information. In summary, it relies on the 'executive thinking' that I mentioned in Chapter 7, and is controlled by the most sophisticated parts of the cortex, also called the executive centres. Throughout the game players receive ongoing information about their rivals' spending decisions, sales, etc, and sometimes, completely unexpected events occur, such as a sudden product recall. Although it is possible to dominate the market in terms of sales, a player can still go bankrupt as a result of reckless overspending. Playing sessions last for an hour at a time, followed by a break of a few hours. In many respects it is like a 'war game' with each player as a military commander trying to defeat opponents.

Our players continued with the game throughout a night without sleep, when their enthusiasm and effort were able to overcome any adverse effects of their sleepiness. But from the next morning and, despite their best efforts, real difficulties became apparent, when they were increasingly unable to comprehend and act on rapidly changing developments. They relied heavily on previous strategies, which were no longer effective or appropriate, and they failed to produce innovative solutions to an increasingly critical situation. They were irritable and began to use more aggressive and exaggerated tactics. Worse still, they became increasingly distracted by irrelevancies and would pursue pointless courses of action. Needless to say, all players eventually went bankrupt and play collapsed in the afternoon. Another group of players, acting as a control group, who slept normally, all successfully played on well beyond this point.

During rest periods, both the sleep-deprived and the sleeping players were tested for their more logical, deductive, and critical reasoning abilities which, unlike the innovative thinking, were unaffected by sleep loss, even towards the end. Other research has shown how remarkably resilient this logical thinking is for up to two days without sleep. Let me explain a little more about this latter type of thinking, which is typical of what is found in IQ tests. This is where all the possible answers and options to a problem are also presented, and it is just a matter of deducing the correct one. For example, in a real IQ test a series of numbers, pictures, or words is given, with all either having something in common or changing in a systematic way. Five possible answers might be shown, with only one being correct. The solution requires a systematic, deductive reasoning—which is the type of thinking not much affected by sleep loss—at least initially. In contrast, executive, innovative, or creative thinking is when there are no potential solutions, often false trails, and irrelevant information, and one has to decide what is relevant and figure everything out from scratch.

Our findings show that people working for extended periods of time, who are required to make innovative decisions, to be flexible in their thinking, and to update their plans in the light of new information, but with little time to ponder on these matters, should avoid sleep loss much beyond one night. It may be a coincidence that renowned disasters or near-disasters caused by human error and concerning nuclear power plants, such as Chernobyl, Three Mile Island, Davis-Beese (Ohio), and Rancho Seco (Sacramento), all occurred early in the morning and involved failure to contain otherwise controllable, but unexpected and unusual, mechanical or control room malfunctions. With all four of these accidents, sleep-deprived but experienced control room managers on nightwork misdiagnosed and failed to appreciate the extent of the fault, and then embarked on courses of action that were inappropriate. They continued to persevere like this, well into the following morning, in spite of clear indications that their original assessment was wrong—they became 'blinkered' or 'tramlined' in their thinking. Of course, it is difficult to say how much of all this could have resulted purely from sleep deprivation rather than from the additional stress and panic.

Sleep deprivation certainly did play a crucial role in the fateful dawn decision to launch the Space Shuttle Challenger, however. The Report of the Presidential Commission[2] on this disaster cited the contribution of human error and poor judgement related to sleep loss and shift work during the early morning hours. Key managers had less than two hours of sleep the night before and had been on duty since 01:00 that morning. They seemed not to grasp the crucial fact that the rocket could not be launched because the outside temperature was too low and might well cause fuel leakage from its tanks—which is exactly what happened. This key point was overlooked among a wealth of distracting information, including trivia that held their interest. The report further commented that 'working excessive hours, while admirable, raises serious questions when it jeopardizes job performance, particularly when critical management decisions are at stake' (p G-5). I cover shift work in Chapter 12.

For crisis management under these situations, a fresh management team must be brought in when the key managers have been awake beyond 24 hours. Despite their best efforts to perform well, their ability to grasp a changing situation, see the 'big picture', and come up with novel solutions would have deteriorated, as would their leadership and communication skills. Whether or not caffeine or more powerful stimulants would reduce the decline in these skills still remains to be seen, because very little relevant research has been done. In the case of caffeine, my own team's findings show that, although it will remove feelings of sleepiness, the poorer executive thinking ability will not be improved by very much. In fact, in the real crises just described, it is likely that liberal amounts of caffeine would have been available to the managers, but seemingly to no avail because the catastrophes or near catastrophes still occurred. As to the minimum sleep length necessary, in an emergency, for an acceptable return of performance to these executive tasks, this must remain an open question for the time being, although I suspect that it will have to be at least 4 hours every 24 hours.

What makes us human?

The executive centres of the brain largely make up the frontal region of the cortex, shown in Figure 3. It comprises about a third of the cortex, is highly developed in humans, orchestrates all of our behaviour, and decides what we are going to attend to and what to ignore. It can rapidly switch to and fro from one activity to another as in 'multitasking', or it can maintain sustained undivided attention to something particularly important, while ignoring competing distractions. Of course, this is probably the seat of our waking awareness and consciousness as philosophers would define it, and the source of what Descartes perceived in '*cogito ergo sum*' ('I think therefore I am'). It is where 'me' largely resides. It draws in the skills of other parts of the cortex as and when required, but in a flexible way (especially in the younger brain), and ensures that all parts of the cortex are 'talking' to each other. In terms of mathematical 'Chaos Theory', the frontal cortex could be seen as a 'strange attractor', in coalescing what goes on in the entire cortex, to create so much variety in our actions. Put simply,

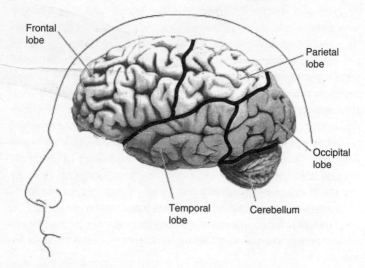

Figure 3 'Lobes' of the human brain—the frontal lobe being the largest.

it is largely the key to the human mind, which is a word that many neuroscientists do not like to use, because 'mind' is seen as too vague and unscientific a term, and largely in the realms of the psychoanalyst and philosopher. So, instead, let us go back to calling it the centre of executive functioning. I should add a reminder, however, that other apes such as the chimpanzee, gorilla, and orang-utan, also have a fairly well-developed frontal cortex, not to the level of ours, but I am sure that they must have minds of some sort!

Although the cortex as a whole works very hard in wakefulness, the frontal area works even harder and, if human sleep is of particular benefit to the recovery of the cortex, as seems to be the case, sleep is probably even more vital here. It is why this area and the behaviours that it controls suffer particularly during sleep loss, even though other regions of the cortex can, to some extent, probably switch in to help out when it begins to fail. Not surprisingly, progressive loss of function of this region, beyond about 30 hours without sleep, begins to turn us into automatons, eventually unable to think for ourselves, as happened with Randy Gardner (see Chapter 4).

So far I have mentioned only some of the behaviours involving the frontal cortex, affected by sleep loss. Here is a recap, including a few of the more important ones:[3]

- Dealing with all types of novelty
- Comprehending and coping with a rapidly changing situation
- Remembering when events occurred
- Remembering very recent events
- Keeping track of events and updating the 'big picture'
- Doing several things at once ('multitasking') by remembering what you are doing, when to shift attention to another event currently being dealt with, and when to return back to the previous task
- Ignoring irrelevant information
- Changing one's plans following new information
- Producing innovative solutions to problems
- Assessing risks and anticipating the range of consequences of an action
- Showing insight into one's own performance

- Having plenty of appropriate words to use for speaking (no paucity of speech)
- Communicating effectively
- Controlling 'uninhibited' behaviour such as irritable outbursts and losing one's temper
- Empathy with other people and detecting subtleties in their behaviour.

Some of these behaviours are particularly interesting, and so let us look at them further, especially as they are seldom mentioned in the context of sleep loss, largely because they are difficult to measure.

Lost for words

Effective verbal communication relies not only on what words we use for speech, but also on the capacity to convey information in a style appropriate to the context of the intended message. The frontal cortex enables us to produce appropriate words to describe complex and changing situations, and this 'verbal fluency' is impaired by sleep loss. There are practical consequences, especially in those situations where sleep-deprived personnel, in control rooms, hospital emergency rooms, and the military, have to communicate about potential crises, etc. A particularly good experimental test of this verbal fluency involves being able to respond rapidly to a common noun, such as 'apple', with as many relevant verbs as possible, such as 'bite, eat, chew, crunch', etc. A series of different nouns (for example, pen, knife, shoe, cup) is given over a short period of five minutes. Adjectives and variants such as 'biting, bitten, bit' do not count of course. Although this task defies the notion that for a test to be sensitive to sleepiness it has to be long, tedious, and dull, this one is the opposite in all these respects, and sleep loss beyond about 30 hours will markedly reduce the number of verbs produced.[3]

Easier to spot is that sleepy speech also becomes less articulate, 'flattened', more laboured, and with longer pauses. Sentences become shorter and we rely more on clichés. There is more mumbling and mispronunciations, with slurring or words run together or in the wrong sequence. What is more, all these impairments are not easily overcome by caffeine or by increased effort to compensate, for example, as happens with the lapses during reaction time testing. It seems that, by about 30 hours without sleep, any 'spare capacity' for the cortex to cope with these deficits, begins to run out.

The first report of these changes in speech intonation with sleep loss was made almost 50 years ago,[4] when the following was noted:

> Alterations in the rhythm, tone and clarity of the subjects' speech were among the most striking observable changes during sleep deprivation. As sleep deprivation progressed, speech usually became slower, softer and contained more unexpected breaks in rhythm. Slurring and softening were often sufficiently marked that the listener could not understand the subject's statements. . . . The usual variation in loudness and pitch was attenuated in most subjects, producing a curious flatness. (p 252)[4]

Despite this common observation, seen more as an aside to the other more measurable findings with sleep loss, no other study except one of my team's has really measured this change.[4] To eke it out we asked our volunteers to read from the short story, 'The Raven', from *Grimm's Fairy Tales*. It is a dramatic tale with much dialogue involving whispering, shouting, and a variable pace to convey slow- and fast-moving pieces of the story. Participants were encouraged to vary pitch and intonation, to act out dialogue, etc, as if they were reading to an audience of young children. By the way, they had already practised on other tales, had overcome any embarrassment, and were comfortable with all this. We also had a control group of similar people who were not sleep deprived. Assessing voices can be a difficult procedure, and we used six independent judges who rated the voice recordings without knowledge of whether or not the speaker was sleep deprived. Intonation, pace, volume, and rhythm of speech were all assessed. In contrast with the exciting end to 'The Raven', the conclusion of my tale is much more prosaic: intonation was obviously impaired by sleep loss, and the judges were very good at spotting it.

Flexibility

Coming up with new ideas and innovative plans is an executive skill that is particularly vulnerable to sleep loss. An excellent test, lasting about 10 minutes, is the 'Tower of London', which is far from dull despite its apparent simplicity. It can easily be constructed and requires only some wood, glue, and a saw to put together, as well as a little paint—all effortlessly done in the garage. The test measures flexibility in thinking, and involves three coloured wooden blocks being moved around on three vertical wooden spindles: one able to hold all three blocks, another two, and the third just one. Blocks are presented in one arrangement on the spindles and have to be moved to another configuration in a minimum number of moves. For example, the three blocks are placed on the longest spindle, in the order blue, green, and red from the bottom to the top. They have to be shifted from spindle to spindle, into the configuration red on blue on the two-block spindle, with green on the longest spindle, by using the minimum of eight moves, and as fast as possible, without mistakes.

There is a series of different starting arrangements and configurations to be achieved, each requiring a different strategy, with the secret of success being to forget completely the way one problem was solved in order to deal successfully with the next. Sleep loss makes the solutions more difficult, because people continue to persist with a previously successful strategy, which will not work again, and somehow they cannot get it out of their mind—that is, they perseverate, and lose the flexibility in dealing with something new. In all, 12 different problems can be generated by this simple test. Perseveration and inflexibility are at the nub of many of the more subtle effects of sleep loss, and this is why I keep the 'Tower of London' as a paperweight on my desk—as that constant reminder that good science can still be done with the simplest of equipment, and that we should not get carried away with hi-tec apparatus, which can be an all-too-costly end in itself.

Another simple, fast-action test showing how perseveration caused by sleep loss leads to hesitation and delay is seen in another, rather strange task involving 'rapid completion of the obvious'. A short, simple sentence is read out quite quickly, but has the last and very obvious word omitted. Without any delay, respondents have to suppress what they are bursting to say and produce an entirely inappropriate word. For example, to the sentence, 'the letter was mailed without a . . .'. The word 'stamp' comes immediately to mind, but 'stamp' has to be suppressed and replaced by a noun that is completely unrelated—such as 'hat'. Another example is, 'he carved the turkey with a sharp ...' but do not say 'knife'—how about 'telephone'? A fully functioning frontal cortex will allow a quick suppression of the obvious word and rapid production of the incongruous one, whereas around 30 hours of sleep loss causes a marked slowing up, with people blurting out the usual (but wrong) word, followed by 'um' and then, with luck, something quite unrelated. The quicker the response and more unrelated this word, the better the score. This test, like the 'verbs to nouns' and the 'Tower of London', is called a 'neuropsychological test' because it is known to tap into the workings of specific parts of the cortex and, in these cases, needs a fully functioning frontal cortex in order to do well.

Gambling and gambolling

This part of the brain also allows us to make rational judgements in risk taking. Sleep loss impairs this ability, to the extent that we are inclined to take more risks. It has not been studied very much in sleepy people, but might help explain why casinos stay open throughout the night, and why gamblers tend to feel luckier as the night progresses. With my colleague, Dr Yvonne Harrison, we explored this with a gambling game (using 'play money'), where players could either gamble and win small amounts, with reasonably good odds of winning, or become 'high-stake rollers' and go big time with bigger bets, greater potential winnings, but being more likely to lose. The aim, of course, was to win as much as possible, with winnings converted into attractive gifts of different values. After a night without sleep our players took greater risks, made more big-time bets, and were more likely to go bust. For the discerning reader who wants to see the night out at the casino, think again—cash in your chips before it gets too late and go home!

Normally, the frontal cortex also tends to dampen down more excitable behaviours, making us more conventional and socially aware of how others see us—which might also explain why sleep loss can make the sleepy gambler less inhibited, take more risks, and become more euphoric and optimistic. I mentioned in Chapter 5 that some people often get a buzz of excitement during a night of sleep loss, with a loosening of social inhibitions, which subdues with increasing sleepiness. Even in more sombre laboratory settings, outbursts of impatience, childish humour, disregard for normal social conventions, and inappropriate interpersonal behaviours have all been described in sleepy participants. This common finding is usually dismissed by experimenters as being of little interest, because they have to concentrate on the seemingly more important measures. Besides, this sort of observation is best left unreported because it suggests that the experiment was getting out of control! In fact, I can find only one written account, which was another aside, again coming from a study from the 1950s, when the investigators reported, 'several [participants] passed through periods of giddiness and silly laughter, like addled drunks, when their behaviour became uninhibited' (p 354).[5] In the real world, and in crises involving sleep loss, euphoria and emotional outbursts will only worsen the ability of people to cope with the situation, and remains a much-neglected topic.

Tedium

The excitement and stimulation of a casino or partying at night are exactly what the sleepy cortex needs to stop us falling asleep. Take the stimulation away and introduce monotony, as happened in those Second World War weary flight crews mentioned in Chapter 7, or when driving in the small hours along a dull and repetitive motorway, as I will be coming to in Chapter 9, and it is a struggle to stay awake. I also mentioned earlier how most laboratory studies of sleep loss, including our own, utilise monotonous tasks to eke out sleepiness, and purposely eliminate all forms of stimulation or other distractions, by seating participants alone in a sound-proofed and visually sterile cubicle so that they can attend fully to the test. Ostensibly, this allows the participant to devote all his or her attention to the tedious task at hand. I would like to return to this theme again, briefly, not only because this situation leads to the 'microsleeps' mentioned earlier, but also because something interesting is happening with regard to 'distractions', which has never really been studied systematically in its own right, even though we know that sleepy people are so vulnerable to distraction. This is largely because the weary frontal cortex can no longer avoid distractions, as it would do normally. Instead, it seeks distraction in an attempt to get new stimulation to enable it to remain awake.

Apart from impaired productivity and more mistakes, sleepiness-related distractions may be of little real harm to someone working in an open office environment, with people talking in the background, telephones ringing, or others constantly walking by. But for those who have to monitor surveillance screens this is a problem, because they might miss important events. Of greater concern is the sleepy train or motorway driver trying to stare ahead, but liable to be distracted by irrelevant but interesting 'rubbernecking' scenes. Worse still, because of the perseveration mentioned earlier, they may dwell on the distraction for longer than usual. Particularly likely to cause distraction is something moving in the 'corner of the eye'—even movement-like activity, such as a bright or flashing light, will have this effect. One can only wonder whether the orange flashing warning lights on broken-down vehicles parked on the hard shoulders of motorways and major highways, in the small hours of the morning, might be causing more harm than good!

Lost time

Memory for time—that is, remembering when something happened, rather than what happened—also tends to rely on the frontal cortex. Again, this was first reported in those 1950s' sleep deprivation studies, when it was noticed that people could remember what they had eaten for meals, but not when it was—for example, 'Did I have that steak and chips for lunch today or was it last night?'. Admittedly these experiments were undertaken in boring surroundings and it is not surprising that the participants found that time passed slowly. However, time for them was 'different', and sometimes it would seem to pass very rapidly. This is another interesting finding that has been largely overlooked until recently, when we used a simple and appealing test in another of our sleep deprivation experiments.[6] This test is also easy to construct, because all that is needed is a few old magazines containing pictures of unknown faces, with 48 different faces in total. To begin with, 12 different faces are presented, one by one, every 4–5 seconds, and the participant is asked to memorise them. Five minutes later, another 12 different faces are shown in the same manner. After a 5-minute further delay, the two sets of faces are shuffled together with 24 more (unseen) faces, making 48 in all. These extra 24 faces are 'foils', given to reduce the effects of guessing. All the faces are now shown one by one and the participants asked: 'Have you seen this face before (yes or no)—if so was it from the first or second set?' Sleep loss has little effect on the first part of the question because people are very good at remembering faces, anyway, and our participants knew which faces they had previously seen. But sleep loss certainly made them forget from which of the two sets of faces these came—that is, they could not remember when they saw them! Similar tests can be done with 48 short, simple, written sentences or abstract shapes, as the outcome with sleep loss is the same.

The big picture

Let me recap on this chapter. Sleepiness feeds on monotony, and the most sensitive laboratory tests of sleepiness maximise this effect by making tests simple, dull, and monotonous. Mild levels of sleepiness can certainly be eked out by such tasks. And, as it is only mild, this sleepiness can easily be counteracted by increased compensatory effort, or by a stimulant such as caffeine. However, all this ignores other, important, and rather fascinating aspects of sleepiness that are not so easy to measure, but are integral to human nature and also very relevant to the real world. More complicated and stimulating tasks are not so affected by mild sleep loss initially, because the inherent interest that they generate encourages more compensatory effort to be applied. This is especially so with well-trained, logical, deductive skills. As to how compensation works, this is a matter for speculation, but it does point to some form of spare capacity in the brain, or back-up system that can be brought in to assist. In contrast, other complex and more demanding 'executive' behaviours, which largely depend on the frontal part of the cortex, seem less able to call upon this spare capacity or reserve, perhaps because there is not enough available. It may also be why applying more effort or drinking coffee is less effective here.

Not only does severe sleep loss make us very sleepy, but also our behaviour gets less 'human', as we gradually turn into automatons, becoming apathetic, losing spontaneity, not knowing where to direct our attention or what to ignore, and having dull and stilted speech. We turn into creatures of routine and are unable effectively to deal with anything new. Personality alters in that we become irritable, and less able to suppress basic emotions or to 'sense' the feelings of others. Arguably, the most subtle role for the frontal cortex is that it enables us to have empathy with other people and to detect nuances in their behaviour. Although this is likely to worsen with sleep loss, it has never been investigated in any systematic way. It might, however, help to explain why sleep deprivation can cause suspiciousness—we fail to see what lies behind what someone is saying or in his or her gestures, which can aggravate interpersonal relationships and non-verbal communication between people. In a crisis situation the sleep-deprived boss may well fail to detect what his juniors are trying to say but are reticent to speak out plainly, or that the overworked sleepy doctor may fail to appreciate what the patient is really trying to say is wrong with him or her.

Loss of sleep often comes from overwork, and other stresses and pressures on our lives, so that some of the apparent effects of sleep loss are not just through lack of sleep, but also from these other stresses. Physical effects or even illnesses attributed to lack of sleep can be caused by this other route. However, it all depends on one's state of mind in dealing with the sleep loss. If we feel quite able to cope with the situation, even seeing it as a worthwhile challenge, the physical effects will be less than if we feel hopeless and no longer in control—it is a mixture of: 'who is in control—is it me or them?' and 'mind over matter'.

A few final points! Most sleep deprivation studies have used young adults, more specifically men, and usually from colleges or junior ranks in the Forces. Hence, much of our knowledge is based on people who are typical of neither the normal population nor more 'senior' decision-makers or commanders who may well be older men and women. Nevertheless, although older people might claim that sleep loss has less of an effect on their sleepiness and abilities than that claimed by younger people, research shows that older people are affected just as badly by sleep loss—which might seem surprising, because older people typically have more experience of sleep loss and might develop some sort of immunity to it. Unfortunately, when sleep loss is repeated as a routine, the more boring the situation becomes, the greater the lack of interest, and the worse the effect, unless all this can be overcome by increasing the incentive to do well. There is a caveat to all this, however, as different coping strategies tend to be adopted. Whereas older individuals are more likely to pace themselves during sleep loss and admit to their deterioration, young adults will usually fight it and are more likely to deny any worsening.

What about natural short sleepers? Are they better able to cope with little or no sleep than long sleepers? As far as we know there is little difference between them in this respect, although there are interesting differences in recovery sleep. Compared with their usual sleep length, long sleepers tend to have less of a rebound increase in sleep after sleep deprivation. Seemingly, their usual sleep is more able to soak up the extra recovery sleep need, whereas short sleepers are already down to their sleep minimum, and recovery sleep has to be added on. More about this in Chapter 17.

Artificial ageing?

Inasmuch as the frontal cortex works the hardest during wakefulness and begins to fail without sleep, there is an interesting parallel with natural, healthy ageing (without sleep loss), because ageing also particularly affects this part of the cortex. This is nothing to do with a lack of sleep in older people—simply that, like any other hard-working mechanism, this part of the brain wears out more quickly with age. Again, with my colleague Dr Yvonne Harrison, we compared the effects of sleep deprivation in healthy young adults with those from two groups of healthy non-sleep-deprived older people with similar educational backgrounds to those of the younger people. One 'older' group averaged 60 years of age and the other, the 'oldest', averaged 73 years. After a good night's sleep and feeling quite refreshed, both the latter groups were given the 'verbs to nouns', 'rapid completion of sentences', and the memory for time (the 'faces') tests. Scores for all three tasks in the older group were similar to those of the young adults, sleep deprived for around 30 hours, whereas, for the oldest group, their scores were the worst. To cut a long story short, it is as if we could simulate natural ageing in young people simply by depriving them of sleep for a night. Had we deprived the younger people of sleep for a longer period, then the further deterioration would probably have reached the level of the oldest group. Even when we gave the young sleep-deprived group caffeine to remove all their feelings of sleepiness, performance on these three tests was still worse than normal, indicating that caffeine and perhaps other stimulants do not really help the sleep-deprived frontal cortex, maybe because it is already working at its best and nothing more can be squeezed out. Of course, recovery sleep fully reverses this deterioration in our young volunteers, but unfortunately, and as one would expect, more sleep for our healthy seniors will not improve matters.

In 1919 the famous German psychiatrist, Dr Ernest Kraepelin, identified a disorder that he called 'dementia praecox' (premature dementia) in young adults. He wrote:

> ... if it should be confirmed that the disease attacks by preference the frontal areas of the brain ... this would agree with the psychic mechanisms which are principally injured by the disease. (p 219)[7]

We now know that in many respects this illness does resemble severe ageing of the frontal cortex, but to a greater extent than is normally found in natural ageing, and certainly far worse than the effects of sleep loss in young people. Nowadays, this disease is often called 'type 2 schizophrenia', which is a more benign type of schizophrenia without the delusions, hallucinatory voices, paranoia, suspiciousness, and hostility—typically known as 'type 1 schizophrenia'. The main symptoms of type 2 schizophrenia include: an inability to focus on relevant issues, paucity in speech, being easily distracted, emotional flattening, lack of spontaneity, and stereotyped thinking— all of which I have mentioned before, but in the context of sleep deprivation in healthy people.

Even at the best of times, these patients do badly on the neuropsychological tests. I must emphasise, however, that sleep deprivation does not cause type 2 schizophrenia; it is just that both situations happen to affect the frontal cortex and there are other symptoms of this illness that neither involve the frontal cortex nor are produced by sleep loss. Moreover, the patients will usually frankly deny that anything is wrong, whereas sleep-deprived people usually know that they are not functioning so well. Interestingly, sleep in these patients is unusual, because it shows little of the deep form of sleep that, in healthy young and old people, is thought to reflect recovery of the cortex, especially in the frontal cortex. More about deep sleep in Chapter 13.

Crashing out

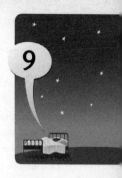

The cost

Sleepiness can be fatal during driving. In fact, this is the most likely reason why sleepiness and sleep loss is harmful to health, and is a topic of much public interest and one where sleep research can be of particular benefit to society. Much of my own work has been in this area and is the reason why this chapter delves into what, at first glance, may seem to be straightforward issues. Until recently, and on dull and monotonous roads, such as UK motorways, US freeways, and European autobahns, many sleep-related crashes were simply attributed to 'driver error' or 'inattention'. It is only in the last few years, with more careful investigations, that it has been realised that there is often more to this inattention than meets the eye, and in the UK, at least, falling asleep at the wheel accounts for around one in five crashes on these dull and monotonous roads. Other apparent causes of crashes, such as tyre 'blow-outs', often turn out to be sleep related, because the blow-out is a 'blow-in' caused by the wheel hitting the kerb or other solid object after the driver has fallen asleep. Sleep-related crashes are almost twice as likely as the 'average' crash to end in death and serious injury, owing to the relatively high speed of the vehicle on impact—there is no braking or swerving beforehand, of course. Apart from the human misery that they cause, the financial cost of these crashes can be huge. For example, following the Selby rail crash, in 2000, where a sleepy driver ran off the road onto a railway track and derailed two trains, resulting in 10 passenger deaths and almost 100 people being seriously injured, the financial liability on the insurance companies was tens of millions of pounds.

Sleep-related truck crashes can be particularly bad as a result of the vehicle's size and momentum on impact—being even more likely to kill the occupants of a struck car. The typical central crash barrier will not deflect or repel a fully laden truck hitting it at about 60 miles (95 km) per hour—which tends to happen when a truck driver falls asleep and ploughs through to collide with oncoming vehicles. Even without fatalities, the UK Department for Transport estimates the average cost of a sleep-related truck crash to be £1.2 (US$2.2) million, including the loss of the truck and its load. Falling asleep at the wheel is also the most likely cause of a truck driver being killed at work, and arguably the most likely cause of someone at work causing a death of another person. Company car drivers are also at risk of having these crashes, not only because of the large annual mileage, but also because they are less likely to pull in for a break or take an overnight stop. Understandably, driving is seen as unproductive time between meeting clients, 'clinching deals', or earning a commission—the quicker the journey can be accomplished, the more time there is to be with the customer. Another vulnerable group are night drivers, including doctors on call, and those driving home at around 6 or 7am after a long night shift.

Unfortunately, the interior designs of modern cars, and especially truck cabs, makes driving very comfortable, so that they are almost 'beds on wheels', with power steering, automatic gears, all controls within easy reach, plenty of sound insulation, a gliding suspension system, and, above all, ergonomically designed seats. Attractive as all this may be for the driver, it may only heighten the risk of driving even longer distances without a break, only to fall asleep at the wheel.

Tell-tale signs

Most of these crashes occur between 2 and 6am, during the daily trough of our body clock (see Chapter 10), in drivers who have had little or no recent sleep, and who probably knew that they should not have been driving then. Besides, drivers who fall asleep at the wheel are aware of sleepiness before the crash and could have stopped beforehand. These are not accidents but easily preventable crashes that cannot be blamed on the '24-hour society', or a sudden and unforewarned 'sleep attack'—the driver is responsible and there is no excuse, as we will see.

Long, undemanding, and monotonous driving, typified by that on motorways, facilitates sleepiness but it does not create it, because one has to be sleepy to begin with. The notion that these roads cause 'highway hypnosis' in an otherwise alert driver, is nonsense, and this is simply a synonym for sleepiness. On the other hand, many of us have experienced 'driving without awareness'—that strange feeling of having driven for the last ten minutes or so with no recollection of knowing where one has been. It is not indicative of falling asleep but usually being on a routine drive and thinking about other things. We can watch TV or read a newspaper 'without awareness', with little subsequent idea of what has been seen or read—not because of dozing off but, really, it was not very interesting and one's mind wanders off to other matters. We are quite able quickly to respond to something new and interesting, or in the case of driving, to that vehicle braking ahead.

Few sleep-related crashes happen in towns or on urban roads because the driving conditions are relatively stimulating and, usually, there is much for the sleepy driver to see and do. In these collisions, the driver typically drifts from one lane to another before running off the road and/or colliding with another vehicle or object. The key sign[1] of an absence of skid marks or evidence of hard braking beforehand is usually because the driver had a 'microsleep' or 'lapse' (see Chapter 7), typically lasting around seven seconds and often much longer. Thus the driver would have seen clearly the point of run-off or the object that he hit (it is usually a he) if he was awake, and could have easily braked or swerved. This is prolonged inattention rather than just a momentary distraction, such as looking out of the side window or adjusting the radio. No one would normally take their eyes off the road for this length of time and, as prolonged inattention points to the driver being unconscious, any sudden illness has to be ruled out before sleep is ruled in. Also, of course, other causes need to be elim-inated, such as mechanical defects in the vehicle, bad weather, poor road conditions, speeding, driving too close, the driver having drunk excess alcohol, taken recreational drugs or even certain medicines, and, occasionally, even the possibility of the driver attempting suicide. Sometimes the vehicle slows down beforehand, because fall-ing asleep produces a general relaxation of body muscles (for example, 'head nodding'), including loss of foot pressure on the accelerator pedal. Whether or not the vehicle actually slows down depends on the strength of the return spring in the accelerator pedal, and if it pushes the relaxed foot upwards.

Although most drivers who are still able to talk after these crashes do not admit to having fallen asleep, or being sleepy beforehand, they are mistaken—I explain why, shortly. Nevertheless, it is surprising the number of drivers, in general, who will freely admit to having felt close to falling asleep at the wheel and having a near miss—some view this almost as a routine hazard of driving and are quite happy to disclose their favourite 'techniques for staying awake'. It is amazing how candid and guiltless many drivers are in telling us their own tricks for staying awake, often enthusiastically exhorting us to try them out as well! Among the most alarming was from a woman with long hair: she would lock her hair in the sunroof of her car, so that when she nodded off the pull on her hair would wake her up. Other recommendations included: removing one's shoes (while still driv-ing) and driving in bare feet, having an elastic band around the wrist with a drawing pin underneath, sucking sliced lemons, moving the driving seat to an uncomfortable position, and, worse still, driving faster. It is an extraordinary attitude to road safety, and I have even met a driver who freely admitted falling asleep at the wheel and who, rather than advocate 'do not drive tired', recommended having a par-ticularly crashworthy car!

Understandably, the dangers inherent in driving encourage sleepy drivers to put a great deal of effort into remaining awake. As a result, falling asleep at the wheel is not the same as when one lies down in bed, expecting to sleep, and falling sharply into obvious sleep. The sleepy driver will fight sleep by winding down the window for cold air, turning up the radio, and using the other favourite tricks just mentioned. As all are conscious acts, it must be self-evident to these drivers that they are sleepy. Such a determination to stay awake causes some sleepy drivers to go into a trance—which is simply a microsleep with the eyes open. This finding is far from new because it was first reported 70 years ago by a Dr Miles, in an article in the magazine, *Scientific American*,[2] where he noted: 'a motorist or anyone may actually be asleep, even if the eyes are seen to be open'. It also throws doubt on the effectiveness of any device for detecting driver sleepiness that depends on the eyes closing.

Response time in applying the brakes in an emergency is commonly thought to be somewhat slower in the sleepy driver, but this is not really the case, because a sleepy driver will respond either almost normally or not at all—which is too late unless he wakes up suddenly beforehand. So, the idea of using some sort of reaction time measure to detect sleepiness in drivers is of little practical use. *'Caveat emptor'* (let the buyer be aware) also applies to various devices claimed to monitor head nodding in sleepy drivers. These have been around in one form or another for many years. Some go over the ear and emit a loud buzz; another is held by the front teeth and, as the jaw muscles relax (when falling asleep), the device falls out of the mouth and its alarm goes off. How one turns it off is unclear, and the thought of the driver scrabbling about trying to retrieve it, with one hand on the wheel, suggests a recipe for disaster. A variant of this ridiculous device involves an inflatable neck collar that is compressed when the head and chin sag, so setting off its alarm—worse still, it can act as a sort of pillow that could even encourage sleep.

Unfortunately for those devices relying on head nodding, and dependent on the position and inclination of the driver's seat, sleepy heads do not always nod forwards—they can just balance upright in that super-comfortable driver seat! Besides, by the time sleepiness gets to this point it is usually too late, because only a second or so may be left before any collision. Much more 'intelligent' systems for identifying driver sleepiness are needed, such as the advisory system for tired drivers (ASTiD[3] in short), which combines information on how well the driver has slept recently, the body's circadian clock and the naturally 'sleepy' times of the day, and whether the vehicle is on a monotonous road. It then detects whether the driver's usual frequent steering corrections become erratic or cease, as happens when sleepiness becomes more profound.

Deadly hours

Apart from the daily peak in these crashes between 2 and 6am, there is another, smaller mid-afternoon surge linked to the natural rise in sleepiness, also caused by the body clock, which is worsened by a poor night's sleep. With my colleague, Dr Louise Reyner, we have been investigating these crashes over several years. What many drivers do not realise is that, considering the few vehicles on the roads in the small hours, the chances of having a sleep-related crash between 2 and 6am are well over 10 times greater than during the early evening, when our body clock is naturally at greater levels of alertness. During the mid-afternoon these crashes are about three times greater than in the early evening.

Various prescribed and 'over-the-counter' (non-prescribed) medi-cines, as well as alcohol and 'social drugs', can also cause sleepiness and, if taken when a driver is already sleepy, will markedly worsen the sleepiness, often to a dangerous extent. Many of us notice that even a small amount of alcohol drunk at lunchtime, well below the legal limit for drivers, can easily 'go to one's head', whereas the same amount taken early evening has no such effect. The reason is that, although many people may not normally have an afternoon surge in sleepiness, this is still a vulnerable time of the day to be sleepy, and anything mildly soporific is more potent at this time. In fact, alcohol at lunchtime is about twice as potent as in the early evening. In both situations the levels of alcohol in the blood are the same. The 'busi-ness lunch' that includes only moderate alcohol consumption, well within the legal driving limits of most countries (and in the UK, within the 'green—all clear' zone on a police breathalyser), presents a serious risk for any monotonous driving that afternoon. As might be expected, this situation is even worse in the small hours of the morn-ing, when driving well beyond bedtime. Recent research coming from France, conducted by Dr Pierre Philip[4] and his team, found that blood alcohol levels as low as one-eighth of the British legal limit and one-fifth of the typical American limit will further impair sleepy driving at these early hours, especially when driving on an empty and mon-otonous road.

Thus, blood or breath alcohol levels can be poor guides to driver impairment at the best of times, and can even worsen sleepiness when these levels have fallen virtually to zero. We have found in our own work that, whereas the alcohol in a pint of beer or a double spirit consumed at 12.30pm has largely disappeared from the blood or breath within three hours, it will still aggravate afternoon sleepiness. Many of us notice this even under safe but mundane circumstances, sitting at a desk, fighting off sleep in the middle of the afternoon, having had only a glass of wine or half a pint of beer that lunchtime.

Much attention has been drawn to studies likening sleepy driving to driving when alert but under the influence of alcohol. For example, a night without sleep is seen to be equivalent to being just over the British legal alcohol limit, and well over the American limit, but without sleep loss. However, the situation is probably worse than this for sleepiness by itself, because the testing sessions used for these comparisons may last for only a short while—not long enough. Whereas alcohol effects may well wear off after a while, with sleepiness it will get worse.

Drivers aged under about 30 years, usually men, are particularly liable to have their sleep-related crashes in the early morning; this results partly from their being the most common group of road users at this time of day. Moreover, they are at a greater risk because younger adults going without sleep experience higher levels of sleepiness than they will usually admit to. Largely out of bravado, they deny that they are likely to fall asleep, claiming to be 'easily able to deal with it', although freely admitting to being somewhat sleepy. More elderly drivers tend to have their sleep-related crashes in the early afternoon, largely because they tend naturally to experience heightened levels of afternoon sleepiness—and, it seems, they are more likely to be out on the road at this time.

The driving and working hours of truck and bus drivers in the European Union (EU), the USA, and Australia are regulated by laws that, unfortunately, pay little regard to the time of day. In the EU, for example, truck drivers can drive for at least four hours continuously without a break, irrespective of the time of day. In the USA the recent changes to 'hours of service rules' for truck drivers still allow up to 11 continuous hours of driving. There is no scientific basis for these being 'safe' lengths of time to drive, especially on monotonous roads and at night. Many early morning sleep-related crashes involving trucks occur within two hours of the journey's start. For example, the driver started work at 4am, and crashed at around 6am when the body clock is still in its daily trough, and despite having had maybe four or five hours sleep beforehand. Many motoring organisations advocate that car drivers take a break around every two hours and it is strange, to say the least, that one 'rule' applies to one type of driver—with the assumption that the professional truck driver, driving a far more dangerous vehicle than a car, is somehow superhuman and can drive for twice as long without stopping.

The EU laws governing truck drivers' working hours require that the driver has a daily rest period normally of ten continuous hours, which is the same for the USA. However, in neither case is there any stipulation that the rest necessitates sleeping. In the USA, the driver may take his rest within the confines of a relatively comfortable sleeper berth, the size of a small caravan, behind the main driving cabin, which is usually very well equipped with waking entertainments. In the EU, playing sport, shopping, family duties, and driving a car all come under this rubric of 'rest', and again there is no instruction to get adequate sleep. Of course, many EU trucks also have sleeping berths behind the driving cab, but these are very cramped and sparse compared with their American counterparts. Besides, sleeping like this at a noisy 'truck stop' or transport café is no substitute for one's own bed.

Sleep disorders?

Driver sleepiness is usually not linked to any sleep disorder, and there is certainly no evidence to show that the most common sleep disorder, insomnia, makes sufferers more likely to have these crashes. Most people with insomnia are not actually sleepy during the day— maybe they are 'tired' but not actually sleepy (I explain why in Chapter 19). Sleep-related crashes are usually caused by healthy people (that is, typically the young men I mentioned) having had little sleep in the previous 24 hours and/or driving during the daily trough of the body clock. Having said all this, however, there is one group of drivers who are prone to suffer from a serious sleep disorder, which can certainly lead to sleep-related crashes—those with 'obstructive sleep apnoea', which is covered in detail in Chapter 21. Briefly, breathing during sleep is periodically prevented by a gagging within the throat, which becomes more likely with obesity, especially with a fat neck and a large belly. In the case of the neck, the weight of the fat further squashes the airway. The tell-tale sign is very heavy ('heroic') snoring, which grossly disturbs sleep, and causes excessive sleepiness during wakefulness. Usually, sufferers are puzzled by this sleepiness, are unaware of any sleep problem, and cannot hear their own snoring— although others trying to sleep nearby are all too aware of it!

Truck drivers tend to eat too much of the wrong foods, especially fried foods, and often at their truck stops or transport cafés. This, together with their rather sedentary lifestyle in sitting in the cab for much of their working lives, means that they tend to become very overweight—hence the apnoea. Truck drivers in the EU drive about 80,000 miles (130,000 km) a year, and about double this amount in the USA and Australia. Much of this is at night, of course, usually when their body clock is at its nadir. If they also have sleep apnoea then they are a danger to themselves and to other road users. Fortunately, there is better news, because most can be treated effectively, virtually overnight, without loss of their jobs or pay. Needless to say, there is a good reason for the screening of truck and other professional drivers, including bus and coach drivers, particularly those who are very overweight and might well have sleep apnoea.

Denial

I would like to return to those healthy young male drivers who are the major cause of sleep-related crashes. They usually deny having fallen asleep, so the evidence pointing to the crash being sleep related has to come from the crash itself. One reason for the denial could be fear of prosecution and loss of insurance indemnity. But it is more likely that the driver genuinely has no recollection of having fallen asleep. Sleep laboratory studies show that people who fall asleep will deny having been asleep if they are awoken within a minute or two of dozing off. Usually, at least two minutes of sleep have to elapse before most of us know that we have been asleep. The reason is that sleep onset makes our perception of both wakefulness and sleep blurred and uncertain, and one has to be well and truly 'out for the count' in order to recognise one's own sleep. As a driver cannot remain asleep for more than a few seconds without having a crash, it is hardly surprising that he does not know that he has fallen asleep.

Although they might be excused for having no knowledge of being asleep, this is no excuse for drivers falling asleep at the wheel, because it is very likely that they were aware of the earlier feeling of sleepiness at the time, even though they may not remember this either. Sleepiness clouds one's memory, and it is common for sleepy drivers to have little subsequent recollection of the events during the period of increasing sleepiness leading up to the crash. This is nothing exceptional, because few of us can remember how sleepy we were before bedtime last night or, more to the point, when this sleepiness first became noticeable. Such recollection becomes even hazier if we try to think back to the previous night. In fact, I bet that you have little idea either! Our brain does not have the capacity to remember such pointless information. The same applies to more benign situations, as in hunger and thirst—we cannot remember either in any detail a few hours after a meal or drink, even though it was usually clear at the time that we were hungry or thirsty. Try to remember how hungry you were before your evening meal last night—when did this begin? How thirsty were you before that first cup of tea or coffee this morning, at breakfast? No idea—you cannot remember—so were you really hungry or thirsty? If not, then why did you eat or drink? Was it just out of habit—surely not? Hardly surprising, then, that drivers who have fallen asleep at the wheel deny being sleepy beforehand.

We have found that, when sleepy drivers are quite honest with us, and are asked after a simulated (safe!) drive whether they can remember being sleepy, they have only a hazy recollection at best, even when they clearly acknowledged earlier, during the driving, that they were sleepy. They may remember saying to us at the time that they were sleepy, but they cannot remember the sensation of sleepiness itself. All in all, then, there is usually little point, after a real sleep-related crash, in asking a driver who has probably fallen asleep at the wheel whether he felt sleepy beforehand or whether he fell asleep. It is even more pointless to ask drivers, when they are being prosecuted in court, to think back often weeks or months after their sleep-related crash, and try to recollect whether they were sleepy at the time. Nevertheless, all this affects legal arguments relating to driver culpability.

Normally, while driving along a motorway in an alert state, drivers are continuously making fine corrective movements to their steering, to keep the vehicle in lane. When falling asleep these corrections cease and the vehicle will drift. With luck the driver soon wakes up, sees what is happening, and makes a violent steering correction. My laboratory has a full-size driving simulator, and we can monitor the progress of sleepiness before drivers fall asleep at the wheel. This is done in various ways: by measuring our drivers' brainwaves (see Chapter 13), by asking them every few minutes how sleepy they are, using the sleepiness scale shown in Chapter 7, and also asking them: 'How likely is it that you will fall asleep in the next five minutes?' This is different from asking 'how sleepy are you?', because we want to know how much insight they have into the risks that they are taking with their sleepiness.

Whenever these drivers drift out of the lane because of sleepiness, we find that they have already stated that they were somewhat sleepy, typically for many minutes beforehand. If they actually reach the stage of falling asleep and running off the road, then they would have already acknowledged a much greater level of sleepiness, such as 'struggling to stay awake', well beforehand. What is surprising is that some of our drivers who admit to being very sleepy continue to drive and then fall asleep at the wheel, having denied that they would fall asleep! They are usually young men who have great faith in their driving prowess and ability to cope with driving while sleepy. This is the real crux of the problem with driver sleepiness—those drivers who know full well that they are sleepy, but think that they are able to stave off falling asleep and continue driving safely.

With the possible exception of certain rare clinical conditions (for example, narcolepsy—see Chapter 14), sleep does not happen out of the blue, spontaneously, from an alert state. There is always a feeling of (often profound) sleepiness beforehand. It is not possible to be alert one minute and asleep the next. A feeling of increasing sleepiness always portends sleep. Sleepy drivers will invariably reach the point of 'fighting sleep', when they will open the window for fresh air, turn up the radio, stretch, and use the various 'tricks' mentioned earlier, which they confidently believe will keep them awake. By the very nature of these acts, drivers clearly demonstrate to themselves that they are sleepy. Why do some sleepy drivers persevere with their driving, beyond the point of fighting sleepiness, and not stop driving? Do they not realise the risks involved? Although sleepiness might cloud their judgement about the extent of the driving impairment, I suspect that they know that their driving is not as good as it should be, but they still consider it to be safe enough. I mentioned, in Chapter 5, that sleepiness can produce feelings of euphoria, which could make some sleepy drivers more optimistic, less cautious, and even reckless with their driving. From whatever perspective one takes, clearly there is a need to educate these drivers that extreme sleepiness is very likely to lead to falling asleep, and a crash. They need continuous reminders—as in the large, prominent signs on UK motorways 'Tiredness kills, take a break'.

Guilty or not guilty?

Given that drivers are aware of sleepiness before having a sleep-related crash, they do have the option of stopping and, if they continue driving, they knowingly take a risk and must accept any consequences of their action. Such a risk is even more foreseeable if they are driving in the small hours of the morning when they are usually fast asleep in bed. However, there have been legal arguments (not in the UK, I should add) that drivers who are falling asleep at the wheel are not able to decide that they are unfit to drive, or know that they are doing anything wrong. In effect, they cannot be held responsible for what might happen, and in legal terms there is no *'mens rea'* (guilty mind), because they are in an 'involuntary state' or experiencing an 'automatism'. If it were also (erroneously) maintained that the driver had no earlier forewarning of sleepiness and just fell asleep at the wheel, then it would be unlikely that he or she would be found guilty of whatever subsequently happened.

Medicolegal issues concerning crashes caused by drivers with diagnosed sleep disorders are complicated.[5] Certainly, a patient with a sleep disorder resulting in excessive sleepiness should not drive until the illness is under satisfactory control. Even if the disorder is not cured, but is successfully controlled, with the doctor declaring the patient 'fit to drive', this does not absolve the patient from the responsibility of ensuring that he or she is fit and able to drive on any particular occasion. A doctor who cautions such a patient about the remaining potential for an increased risk of sleepiness is safeguarding both the health and life of that patient, and the safety and lives of other road users. Moreover, it would be prudent for the doctor to write in the patient's notes that this cautionary information was given, because if this patient subsequently caused a sleep-related driving crash then, in the UK, it is quite possible that this driver could still be prosecuted. This is because driver guilt, *mens rea,* could well be established and, to say the least, it would be unfortunate for the doctor if the patient then tried to pass the blame on to the physician, who unwittingly may have just said to the patient: 'You're now fit to drive.' On the other hand, it could be argued that this driver, having been treated, is still liable to fall asleep more quickly than healthier drivers and has less forewarning of sleepiness—in which case, he or she was probably not fit to drive after all!

Practical countermeasures

In pressing on with their journey, too many unwitting sleepy drivers resort to opening the window or air vents, believing that a blast of cold air into the face will do the trick, or even turning up the car radio/tape player. Neither method is very effective, as Dr Reyner and I found, because both provide only temporary benefit, maybe for about 10 minutes, which at best allows a little more time for drivers to find and stop at a suitable place to park and take their break. Listening to the radio while driving under these conditions, or rather attempting to listen to the radio, can even worsen the situation, because it can distract sleepy drivers from being so aware of their sleepiness and poor driving.

So, take a break and do what? 'Fresh air' and a brisk walk around a stopping or service area, often recommended by driving organisations, are fairly useless methods for overcoming sleepiness—again, lasting maybe for 10 minutes or so before sleepiness returns.

Although heavier exercise—for example, a 10-minute jog—can certainly perk one up for a while, not only is it impractical, but the greater feeling of relaxation that comes after this type of exercise only worsens the sleepiness. Obviously, the best method is to take a nap. Four minutes is the minimum for any benefit at all, whereas naps beyond 20 minutes can be counterproductive because they develop into a more substantial sleep, leading to difficulty in waking up, and a feeling of inertia and 'thick-headedness'. A 15-minute nap is just about right, and the phone or other alarm should be set for this period. A full-blown, 'out-for-the-count' sleep is not essential unless there has been excessive sleep loss, in which case one should not be driving at all. Given that most cars and trucks have very comfortable driving seats, these are ideal for a nap—perhaps too much so if one happens still to be driving. As napping is not always safe from the perspective of personal safety, a safe place must be found and the doors locked.

The next best method for alleviating sleepiness is caffeine, as in coffee or other caffeinated drinks, such as 'functional energy drinks'. Caffeine is a safe drug in moderation,[6] with very few adverse effects, certainly at a dose of 150 milligrams, which is the amount that we recommend, and equivalent to about two average cups of coffee or a can or two of these particular drinks. Unfortunately, coffee does vary considerably in caffeine content, and one cannot tell how much caffeine is present from the coffee's taste, colour, or indeed the price—be warned! This amount (150 milligrams) of caffeine is effective for moderate levels of sleepiness, but of little help if there has been too much sleep loss. As caffeine takes around 20–30 minutes to have its effect, here is the opportunity to take the nap. So, do not nap before the coffee, but do it the other way round—drink the coffee and then use the 20- to 30-minute 'window of opportunity' for a nap—to allow the effects of both to kick in together. We have shown this to be a very effective combination. Our findings with caffeine and naps are the basis for the recommendations for dealing with driver sleepiness, to be found in the UK *Highway Code*—the guide to good driving, issued by the UK Department of Transport to all new drivers.

Drivers should not resort to higher or repeated doses of caffeine on a long journey, because this implies that they are too sleepy anyway, and should not be driving at all. Easier said than done, of course, as the high incidence of sleep-related crashes in the early morning suggests otherwise. Nightshift workers driving home at around 7am, especially after the first night on this shift, have usually had little sleep during the last 24 hours, and should consider alternative transport. However, 150 milligrams of caffeine will certainly help here, but it has to be taken at least 20 minutes before clocking off and, with such a high degree of sleepiness, will be effective for only about half an hour afterwards. Some nightworkers are reluctant to drink this amount of caffeine just before going home, because they worry that it might prevent them from sleeping soon after getting home. However, as we see in Chapter 11, sleeping so soon after a nightshift is not really such a good idea if another nightshift is to follow. Delaying this sleep to later in the day, perhaps with the aid of that caffeine, will help you to cope with the next night.

Greater awareness

These dreadful crashes can be reduced through a greater awareness by drivers and employers of the danger of driving while sleepy, and that such driving behaviour is unacceptable, particularly to other road users. No employer would give their employee alcohol over the legal driving limit, and then allow them to clock off and drive home. The level of driving impairment at 7am, having had no sleep, is worse than being over the British legal drink driving limit, and well over the limits in the rest of Europe and in the USA. So why allow the same thing to happen to a sleepy individual after a nightshift, when he is even less fit to drive? Work and other time schedules ought to be planned so as to minimise exposure to prolonged driving under monotonous conditions during the more vulnerable times of the day and night. The best and most accurate information that drivers have at their disposal about their state of sleepiness comes from their own self-awareness of it. What many drivers fail to appreciate is that sleepiness portends sleep, which can appear more rapidly than they realise, especially if the driver has reached the more profound stage of fighting off sleep and utilising self-demonstrable acts such as opening the window—at which point they should consider what it might be like for their families if they were to complete their journey in a hearse.

10 Time of life

Body clock

Our lives are very much influenced by our body's circadian clock, which affects the timing of sleep and the daily rhythm of alertness, body temperature, and many other functions. In fact, body temperature is the best measure of this clock, because the two are very closely linked. Body temperature and alertness are normally at their daily lowest around 2–6am and at their highest around 6–8pm. The changes in alertness are seen in Figure 4, where alertness rises fairly quickly around the normal wake-up time, at about 7–8am, followed by a levelling off and, often, a small trough or 'dip' around mid-afternoon. There is a final rise to the evening peak, and then a fairly rapid fall up to bedtime and beyond. Whereas the 24-hour change in

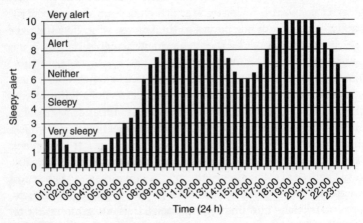

Figure 4 Alertness over the 24-hour day.

alertness is large, that of body temperature is fairly small—only about 0.7°C from peak to trough.

The night-time drop in body temperature does not alter much whether we are asleep or happen to stay awake, because it is not really under the control of sleep itself, but, rather, of the body clock, which is somewhat independent of sleep. For example, delaying sleep to the following morning will reduce the morning rise in body temperature by only a little. Thus, the circadian rhythm, as reflected by body temperature and feelings of sleepiness or alertness, remains fairly stable, with or without sleep, and is slow to change when sleep is moved to a different time of day—which is a problem for the shift worker or time-zone traveller.

The circadian clock naturally runs a little slower than 24 hours, somewhere between 15 and 40 minutes longer than 24 hours—let us say 24.5 hours. However, it keeps better time than this largely through registering daylight, artificial light, and other regular environmental time cues. This particular light detection comes via special, 'non-seeing' cells in the eye, which can remain intact even in blind people. Unfortunately, for those with the most severe eye damage, even these cells are lost, which can lead to ill-timed and irregular sleep patterns.

For most mammals, sunrise and sunset are the clock's main synchronisers, whereas, in the modern world of electric lighting, our clock is not so dependent on daylight and darkness, but artificial light, and even less evident but regular daily cues such as mealtimes, morning wakening by an alarm clock, and perhaps even the daily watching of a regular TV show! If all these time cues are removed, for example, by keeping someone in an artificial environment under constant and subdued light, without watches, clocks, radios, TVs, etc, the body temperature rhythm 'free runs' at its natural 24.5 hours, and will continue to do so until it is re-set by those time cues. For example, after a month of free running, the temperature clock will be about half a day behind real time. Although the timing of sleep is normally closely linked to this temperature clock, as we will see shortly, the two are not exactly 'bed partners', and can go their separate ways as happens under these free-running conditions. Here, sleep breaks free of this clock, which ticks on at its 24.5 hours, whereas sleep becomes erratic, sometimes with over 30 hours between periods of sleep, when sleep length itself can also vary considerably.

Why nature has given us our body clock is not exactly clear, and perhaps in order to understand it we must go back to prehistoric times, when we had no other clocks and relied on the sun for all light. Inasmuch as our internal clock pre-empts each part of the day, it ensures that sleep, wakefulness, alertness, and other various body changes will be at their most suitable levels. For example, at the end of a busy day of simply surviving, our ancestors would be sleepy, and the daily boost alertness at this time, provided by the body clock, could prolong the 'working day' and a safe return home. The body clock also anticipates morning waking by 'cranking us up' beforehand and helps curtail the night's sleep.

Inadequate sleep at night will shift the circadian rhythm of alertness downwards, as shown in Figure 5. The poorer sleep is, the greater the shift and, particularly, the deeper the afternoon dip, which eventually becomes a chasm. Nevertheless, even after the worst of nights, alertness still picks up for a while in the early evening.

The topic of clocks and the struggle of staying awake at night allow me to digress for a moment and recount the origins of the saying,

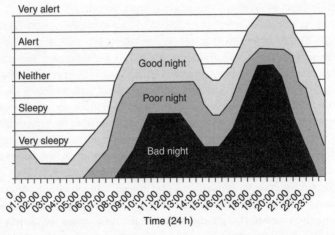

Figure 5 Daytime alertness after a good, poor, or bad night's sleep.

'saved by the bell', originating around 150 years ago, when a guard on night sentry duty at Windsor Castle, near London, was charged with the serious offence of falling asleep at his post. The soldier denied this by claiming that he heard the church bell strike 13 times at midnight. No one believed him at first until it was found that a cog in the bell mechanism had slipped and it had indeed struck 13 times. Much press coverage ensued, and 'saved by the bell' was the oft-quoted story caption.

Sleep time

Excluding the alarm clock, kids, and postman, the length of our night's sleep and when we wake up in the morning depend on both the length of prior wakefulness and the influence of the body clock. Of course, the longer one is awake the more we sleep, which is fairly straightforward, except that there is a diminishing return whereby doubling a period of wakefulness does not double the length of sleep but, rather, only increases it by about a half—I come to this in Chapter 17. To help explain how sleep and the body clock interact, I liken wakefulness to water pouring into a bath, at a fairly constant flow. The rising bathwater reflects lengthening wakefulness and an increasing need for sleep. Pulling the plug corresponds to going to sleep and the initial intense rush of water represents more intense sleep (that is, 'deep' sleep). With the fall in the bathwater, the outflow slows down, eventually to a trickle, and we wake up. If the bath was really full, say after 24 hours of filling, without a night's sleep, the greater would be the initial rush of water (increased deep sleep) and the longer the bath would take to empty (longer sleep). To explain the involvement of the body clock with sleep, I will concentrate on the bath's plug hole, because its width varies according to the time of day, independently of the amount of water in the bath. In simple terms, the plug hole normally widens at around 4–6am, for a few hours, to let out even more water and hasten emptying—and the end of sleep.

For most of us, sleeping is a regular process: same bedtime at night, same length of wakefulness, and, after a normal amount of sleep, our metaphorical bath is just about empty at 7am anyway, regardless of the size of the plug hole. Not so, however, if one is late to bed, because water is still in this bath at 7am, but the widening plug hole will drain the bath much more rapidly, and sleep length will be shorter than usual, even though wake-up time will be delayed somewhat. No sleep at all that night and sleeping in the morning? The extra high water means more sleep than usual, but that gaping plug hole causes the water to leave more rapidly, with the net effect that sleep is shorter during the day. This interaction between sleep 'pressure' and the body clock helps to explain why nightshift workers tend to sleep only five to six hours during the morning if they are not used to sleeping by day. Of course, my bath is only a superficial account of how the body clock and sleep 'pressure' interact, and sleep research owes much credit for the real explanation to Professor Alexander Borbély, from Zurich University, who has pioneered this work in the form of the 'two-process model' of sleep regulation.[1]

Larks and owls

The body clock varies somewhat between people, in the timing of the daily peak and trough, with some of us being 'larks' and others being 'owls'. The lark, or 'morning type' is an earlier riser than the owl or 'evening type', who stays up and goes to bed later. Their sleep lengths are about the same, although larks feel at their daily best in the morning, are able to eat a hearty breakfast, and are often the life and soul of the breakfast table, unlike owls who cannot face more than a slice of toast for breakfast, are rather grumpy then, and best left alone. The tables turn at night when the lark starts sinking fast at around 9pm and is usually out for the count by 10-ish, when the owl is ready to go and take to the wing so to speak.

These are the extremes, because most of us lie somewhere between being an owl and being a lark. About 20 per cent of adults are either true owls or true larks, about 40 per cent are neither one nor the other, and the remainder are either moderate larks or moderate owls. To some extent there is a hereditary aspect to being a lark or owl, but this is not the only effect, especially as older age naturally turns us into more of a lark, whereas young adults tend to be more owl-like, being at their most 'owlish' at around 20 years of age. Interestingly, owls are better at training themselves to become larks, if they so wished, whereas larks are less adaptable and less able to cope with enforced changes to their body clock, as happens with shift work and jetlag. Moreover, as ageing moves us into the domain of larks, this is one reason why older people are less able to deal with shift work.

The good news for larks is that they may well have an advantage over owls, because there could well be some truth in the sayings, 'early to bed, early to rise makes one healthy, wealthy, and wise' and 'the early bird catches the worm'. I do not know about wealth, wisdom, or worms, but there is evidence that the lark lifestyle produces a better daytime mood, making us feel happier and more positive about life. Maybe larks do achieve more than owls, whereas owls have to get their kicks by having a more exciting night life and, according to Ambrose Bierce, the American wit and writer, 'dawn is when men of reason go to bed'.[2]

At the end of this book is a short version of a well-known owl–lark questionnaire. I developed it with my colleague, Dr Olov Östberg, and in its longer form it is still used by sleep researchers world wide, translated into numerous languages.

In the dark of the night

Once, many fish and some reptiles had a transparent area in the centre of their skulls, below which was a crude eye-like structure. Its function was to detect daylight and darkness, and in doing so it probably helped regulate the animal's body clock. This third eye may also have caused changes to skin colour, darkening it by night and lightening it by day—probably for camouflage. The lamprey is a primitive fish that still has it as a sort of functioning eye. One of the few land animals retaining this eye is the New Zealand Tuataras lizard (*Sphenodon* species) also renowned for its 100-year longevity. Nevertheless, we humans have not actually lost this organ because, over the last few hundred million years or so, it has evolved into a somewhat different structure now found deep within the brain, known as the 'pineal gland'—sometimes still loosely called our 'third eye'. Its presence in the human brain was first recorded some 2,300 years ago by the scholar Herophilus, who believed it to be a valve regulating the flow of '*spiritus animus*' (animal spirit), essential to the development of the human intellect.

Although not an eye, this gland is influenced by light from the eyes, as the French philosopher Descartes correctly surmised in 1662; perhaps not so correctly, he also believed it to be the seat of the soul. Until the 1950s, medical textbooks simply regarded it as a useless vestigial organ within the human brain. The breakthrough began in the late 1950s when it was discovered that, in frogs, the pineal organ produced a hormone, originally called 'yalin', because the discoverers were working at Yale University. Subsequently it was renamed 'melatonin', because it controls pigmentation in the frog's skin, in cells already known as 'melanocytes'. Today, we know that melatonin is abundant in the pineal gland of adults who are young to middle aged, and acts as a key mechanism through which light from the eyes helps set the circadian clock, not only for us but also for other mammals. In elderly people the pineal gland becomes calcified and less functional, and has a diminished melatonin output, which can lead to the weaker ('flatter') circadian rhythm commonly found in this group of people. We owe much of our more recent knowledge about the pineal gland and melatonin to Professor Josephine Arendt at Surrey University.[3] Melatonin is the 'hormone of the night' because it is released into the bloodstream during darkness, although this is not caused by sleep itself, because this output is maintained at night in nocturnal mammals and in night-shift workers. For us, melatonin levels are roughly the reverse of the daily temperature rhythm, reaching a night-time peak at around 4am, when the body temperature is at its lowest.

The pineal gland also allows the brain to register the seasonal changes in daylight and darkness, and in doing so helps to control seasonal reproductive cycles in many animals, such as sheep. It may well influence the human menstrual cycle, but this aspect of its function is still not fully understood. Melatonin is also important to the infant mammal, because relatively large amounts slow up growth and low levels speed it up—again on a seasonal basis. In the summer when food and light are plentiful, with melatonin suppression, there is a growth spurt, whereas, in the winter, growth slows down largely as a result of the longer and larger night-time melatonin release and the relative shortage of food. We do not know whether this aspect of its function is also relevant to children.

The pineal gland and its release of melatonin are not the source of the biological clock, because the latter resides elsewhere in the brain, deep behind the eyes, in the suprachiasmatic nucleus, known as the SCN. However, the pineal gland is linked to it, and we might consider its release of melatonin as a sort of regulator for the SCN, which is able to re-set the timing of the clock, rather like moving the hands as opposed to interfering with the clock's mechanism.

Although the surge in melatonin can still be found at night in nightshift workers, for those working under fairly bright artificial light, the surge is suppressed by this light. As melatonin also has a mildly soporific effect, suppression of this surge can improve night-time alertness (bright light can also have a more 'psychological' alerting effect as well). The manipulation of night-time melatonin levels by judicious use of light and/or the aid of melatonin tablets will also modify the timing of the circadian clock. These alerting or clock-shifting effects of artificial light depend on four factors: whether it is similar to daylight in its whiteness (spectral quality) and brightness (lux) and for when and how long one is exposed to the light. For example, 2500 lux, which is about a quarter of the brightness of an average overcast day, given for 2 hours from around 2am, will completely suppress melatonin output and improve alertness, whereas more typical indoor levels of about 300 lux, given for 30 minutes, will have only a limited effect. I should add that white light with a slight blue tinge seems to be the most effective in these respects.

Although melatonin can produce drowsiness, this is nothing like that from a true sleeping tablet, and its real effect is with the timing of the body clock. Remember, melatonin output is suppressed by bright light and one is the antithesis of the other. For example, bright light beginning at dusk, to suppress melatonin, will delay body time, although this will not be dramatic at first, because a few nights of this procedure are needed for any substantial change. On the other hand, bright light given just after the usual trough of the body clock, at 6am, will quickly hasten the natural decline of melatonin at this time, and trick the body clock into thinking that it is later in the morning than is the case. In effect, this shortens the ensuing day (provided that bright light is avoided at dusk), and the subsequent evening's rise in melatonin will be earlier, bringing forward bed-time drowsiness. This is not a quick fix for people with insomnia, however, because there is usually much more to insomnia than problems with the body clock (see Chapter 20).

I have been labouring somewhat over melatonin and its effects, because this substance is becoming very popular in a synthetic form, easily taken as a tablet for self-treatment of jet lag and to help night workers to adjust to the shift regimen. It usually comes in 3 milligram tablets, which can all too easily be bought from any drug store in the USA, although it is not readily available in the UK, where it is difficult to obtain even with a doctor's prescription unless there is a medical disorder. The reason for this difference is that, in the USA, the authorities view it as a form of food, not subject to stringent drug testing, which is the exact opposite for the UK where it is viewed as a drug. It is fairly safe but, as pharmaceutical companies are not really interested in it (they cannot patent melatonin because it is a natural substance), the necessary drug testing has not been undertaken to allow it to be sold in the UK. Instead, many travellers simply buy their supplies in American drug stores, or over the internet—but the purity and strength of the melatonin can vary considerably, so, beware. Again I must emphasise that melatonin tablets and bright light do not mix when used at the same time.

Melatonin tablets taken a few hours before the desired bedtime (ideally at dusk) can be very helpful to blind people whose circadian rhythms are seriously disrupted, for the reasons that I explained above. However, this treatment (which can be prescribed in the UK) works for only about half of these people. Maybe the failure, here, is because their body clocks have been out of control for too many years. Whether or not melatonin should be given to children who are blind or have the 'delayed sleep phase syndrome' (see Chapter 22) remains questionable, because there is a possibility that this hormone might affect puberty.

Melatonin tablets in low doses (for example, 3 milligrams) should not interfere with the menstrual cycle or fertility, if taken for only a few days at a time. It is more likely, however, as the menstrual cycle is also linked to the 24-hour body clock, that making one's body clock more regular can improve an irregular menstrual cycle (that is, dysmenorrhoea), but very high doses of melatonin do inhibit ovulation. There are claims that melatonin might be of benefit in the treatment of breast cancer, in slowing tumour growth. Moreover, it has also been claimed that bright light at night may speed up this growth, because it causes suppression of melatonin output, as happens during short summer nights and with nightshift workers, but such a connection between these events is tenuous.

Ebb and flow

Finally, I would like to return to why our circadian clock seems naturally to want to run somewhat slower than 24 hours when all cues to time are removed. Some believe the culprit to be the moon, and I will explain why this is probably not the answer, albeit an attractive one, although it could be a part answer. Clearly, for all living organisms our circadian clock originated from the rotation of the Earth in relation to the sun and the daily appearance of sunlight. Whereas, for us, the sun is probably the only celestial object affecting our clock, for animals and marine plants living in tidal zones, the tides, or rather the gravitational pull of the moon on the sea to create the tides, has another influence on their circadian clocks because this tells them when food will be available. Some researchers have even argued that, because at least some of our early human ancestors lived by estuaries, our body clock might still be under some sort of rudimentary influence from the moon and tides. But this cannot account for why our body clock is naturally disposed to run roughly between 15 and 40 minutes beyond 24 hours, because, if the moon were having a major effect, this daily delay should be longer, averaging 52 minutes. One problem with pursuing this idea about the moon's influence is that its gravitational and tidal effects on the Earth are not consistent from day to day, but vary systematically.

Whereas the Earth rotates relative to the sun every 24 hours, the moon itself rotates around the Earth every 27 days, 7 hours, and 44 minutes, and in the same rotational direction as the Earth. The upshot of this is, time wise, that the moon falls behind the Earth's rotation and is why the appearance of the moon in the same spot of our sky is delayed between 10 and 90 minutes (averaging 52 minutes) daily. This variation is because the orbit of the moon around the Earth is elliptical (as well as tilting in a systematic way). The overall effect can easily be seen in 'tide tables', giving the varying day-to-day lags in high and low tides. It also means that the moon's orbital speed, distance (apparent 'size'), and gravitational pull on the Earth all vary accordingly.

Although 'sheer lunacy' might well be your appropriate response to any apparent lunar effect on our circadian rhythms, one could argue that for about 12 days per month the tidal delay is in the region of 12–40 minutes per day, rather like that of our circadian clock. But, of course, for the rest of the month the tidal delay goes well beyond this limit!

Time travellers

Eight versus twelve

About one in six working adults is a shift worker of one sort or another, and on various shift patterns. It takes about 10 days of continuous nights for the body clock and sleep to become fully adapted to night work, sleeping normally by day. Unfortunately, this is impractical for all except those who enjoy being on permanent nights. One alternative is for a rapidly rotating shift system, with no more than two, perhaps three, successive periods on any one shift. The body clock cannot possibly adapt to this and simply gives up doing so, staying where it is, and one copes as best as one can. Until recently one of the most common shift patterns was an eight-hour, rapidly rotating shift system of 'earlies' (starting about 6am), 'lates' (2pm), and nights (10pm), entailing two or three periods on each shift. It has the advantage not only of allowing for some additional overtime, but of being able to incorporate at least 24 hours (including a good recovery sleep) for a changeover from one shift to another.

A slower rotation on each of these three shifts—for a week or so at a time—does allow for some adaptation of the body clock, but this is of little real help, and generally means that, on days off, the body clock just flips back to its normal state and one has to start that adaptation process all over again when returning to the next shift. Ideally, eight-hour shift systems should rotate in a forward (that is, clockwise) direction—for example, in the direction: earlies, lates, and nights. The reverse direction is harder to cope with, because this 'compresses' the day on changeover, whereas the body clock is better able to deal with extending the day, as happens with the clockwise direction. This principle also applies to jetlag, as will be seen. So, after a week on an

113

early shift, when some adaptation has taken place, it is better to go on lates rather than nights, especially as the time off between the changeover will probably be longer compared with the less time (for example, 16 hours) provided when shifting backwards.

One disadvantage of the 8-hour rotating system, whether rapid or slow, is that around five sessions have to be worked (for a 40-hour week) before any extended days off can be taken, unlike the increasingly attractive 12-hour shift system (for example, 7am to 7pm) when the shifts are repeated usually for only three nights or perhaps four days in succession. Then, the changeover usually comes with three or even four days off (especially following the night shifts), which is very popular with the workforce and seems a good idea. Unfortunately, three 12-hour nights in succession can be so exhausting that the first day off (or more) is almost spent in convalescence, or rather in recovery and, contrary to popular belief, this shift system is probably not so worthwhile, especially as there are other disadvantages. It almost goes without saying that 12 hours of dull and monotonous night work can be a recipe for disaster if the job cannot be made more flexible and interesting in some way.[1] Even so, most people cannot sustain 12 hours of work through the night and most will be struggling to stay awake by around 4am, when their output will deteriorate markedly, and thereon for the ensuing last few hours of the shift. This is even more evident on the first night of a 12-hour shift, because usually by the end of it people have probably been awake for 24 hours, when they are neither fit nor safe to drive home afterwards, as I have already cautioned. Indeed, 12-hour shifts are already too long for overtime to be added, because people must have at least 12 hours between shifts to allow for travel to and from work, as well as for some reasonable recovery.

A few organisations work 10-hour shift systems as a compromise between 8 and 12 hours, but this is difficult to schedule and involves overlap in shifts, although the latter can be useful. Probably the worst shift patterns are 'split shifts'. Although this may total 10 hours of paid work per shift, there is an extended break, often lasting 4 hours or so (often without pay) in the middle of two 5-hour work periods. This system is mostly found in the catering industry with, for example, staff working lunch times and evenings, and the afternoon off, but too short a period to go home and rest.

Naps

Day sleep following all types of night-shift systems is usually lighter and shorter than usual, as described in Chapter 10, because the body clock is still on its daily rise in the morning when most night workers want to sleep. The five hours of daytime sleep, which is often typical here, is insufficient. Of course, there are other reasons for daytime sleep to be curtailed: noise, too much light, and family commitments such as having to pick the kids up from school. All this makes it sensible for people on 8- and 10-, and definitely on 12-hour night shifts, to be encouraged to take one or two short naps, lasting for no more than 15 minutes (otherwise there will be too much unwanted grogginess) during the meal or rest breaks. A nap will certainly help in coping with the last few hours of this shift as will fairly frequent breaks, ideally for 5–10 minutes, about every 2 hours.[1] Now, it might seem to an employer that all these rests and naps make an idle workforce, reduced work output, and lost profits. Wrong—these interludes will boost output during the actual work period, reduce the risk of accidents, make a happier workforce, and even reduce sick leave.

As they are so sleepy, many people coming home from the night shift go straight to bed. However, better sleep will be gained if it is taken later in the day, especially if there is another night shift to follow. The nearer this sleep is to the next shift, the less will be the sleepiness during the shift. In this respect, another advantage of allowing a nap or two in the night shift, and especially if it is a 12-hour shift, is that people will not be so sleepy going home and will be better able to keep going for a few more hours, at home, before going to bed. Having caffeine about 20–30 minutes before the end of this shift, to increase alertness on the way home, will further help to delay that sleep.

Enlightenment

Bad morale among shift-workers generates costs that do not show on budgets, but the expense soon piles up. An astute manager realises that looking after the health of a workforce should be judged by outcomes rather than price—poor 'presenteeism' costs industry more than absenteeism. Whereas a well-managed shift system not only reduces absenteeism and sickness, staff turnover, compensation claims, and 'lost time' incidents, if it is too well managed people will be much fitter and tempted to undertake other 'moonlighting' jobs during their days off. Whatever benefits are gained may simply be used to facilitate another job—then to rebound on the shift.

'Earlies', or day work in general, ought not to begin before 6–7am because this usually means that people have to get up particularly early and probably have had inadequate night sleep. Besides, they may well be travelling to work, when the body clock is still in its trough. On the other hand, too late a morning start, especially on a 12-hour system, can mean difficulty in getting back home on public transport in the evening.

Bright indoor light at night increases alertness, as mentioned in Chapter 10. There is a possible drawback, however, because one problem is that the glare can be uncomfortable; therefore a balance has to be reached with the brightness—not too bright but enough to reduce the melatonin levels. A compromise for the night worker is lighting at about 1500 lux, typical of an office with a window letting in normal daylight. As I also mentioned, a slight blue tinge to the white light can be better still, because the light-sensitive mechanisms in the eye, linking to the melatonin release, are most receptive to this type of light.

Shift work is unnatural, and leads not only to disruption of the body clock, sleep difficulties, and sleepiness at work, but also to headaches, indigestion, constipation, and the additional strain of family and social disruptions. Rather than nap, many people rely on a few coffees throughout the night, which are harmless and helpful, but some night workers depend too heavily on this caffeine and overdo it—needing sleeping tablets to unwind, relax, and sleep when they get home. Here, it is likely that a higher than normal dose of sleeping tablets will be needed to help with daytime sleeping, leading to a hangover at work, more caffeine, and development of a vicious cycle that could result in illnesses of one sort or another. It is better simply to take those short naps during breaks, perhaps with modest caffeine in between.

Coping

So far, I have not used the term 'tiredness'. I see it generally describing the feelings of being worn out, 'heavy limbed', listless, with loss of interest, difficulty in getting going, and feeling rather miserable. I explain this more, in Chapter 18, but suffice it to say that this tiredness is not necessarily the result of sleep loss and differs from 'sleepiness', which is simply an increased propensity to sleep. For many people, the term 'fatigued' is synonymous with being tired, as well as with being sleepy, all of which can be very confusing. However, 'fatigue' really relates to the effects of prolonged physical or mental work, rectified by rest or a change of scene, but not necessarily by sleep. I do not want to delve further into the semantics of all these words, now, but merely want to say that shift work can produce all three: sleepiness, tiredness, and fatigue. All can interact with each other and lead to that other problem, 'stress', a difficulty in coping with shift work and, again, maybe leading on to illnesses of one sort or another. This is especially so if the shift-work schedules are poorly designed, with long working hours and inadequate rest days—thus aggravating the demands of both work and home. Although a supportive family and plenty of quality time spent with them and friends can be of enormous benefit, a shift worker who has a disrupted home or social life may well feel isolated, moody, or depressed—thus further affecting health and work.

There are two main health problems linked to long-term exposure to shift work: stomach (peptic) ulcers and cardiovascular complaints (including heart disease). Stress may well be behind both, although there are other, indirect and undesirable effects of shift work, such as a poor diet (too many snacks), too little exercise, and a greater likelihood of smoking. Nevertheless, when all these effects are discounted, these two health problems remain, albeit to a lesser extent.

Professor Torbjorn Åkerstedt from the Karolinska Institute, in

Stockholm, is an eminent sleep researcher who has convincingly shown us how sleep—its length, quality, and when it is taken during the shift regimen—plays such a crucial role in the ability to cope. Two of his recent studies are particularly important because they have looked at long-term health effects[2] and fatal occupational accidents[3] in shift workers. The first located 169 pairs of identical twins (out of almost 50,000 surveyed), aged over 65 years (that is, they had retired), where one of each pair had spent many years (average of 12 years) as a night worker, and the other only as a day worker. 'Night' twins were almost twice as likely to report impaired health and three times more likely to have sleep problems. Of course, it would be unwise to blame the night work for all of this, but it is suggestive. The second study was a bit grimmer, and over 20 years followed up almost 48,000 people who were regularly interviewed about their health, sleep, work practices, etc. Of those studied 160 subsequently died at work in an accident of their own making. Their previous interviews were checked, and the most salient predictors were not age, education, socio-economic group, workload, overtime, or being a manual worker, but being male, having difficulties in sleeping, and working nights.

I mentioned earlier that 'larks', as opposed to 'owls', can cope fairly well with early shifts, whereas owls may have some difficulty. Nevertheless, owls still do better with shift work overall. This is partly to do with age, because adults aged under 40 years tend to be more owl-like, whereas older individuals become more like larks. Older shift workers (usually over 50 years) not only have more difficulty in coping with the disruptions, but may also have greater problems with sleeping by day. For different reasons, teenagers can also have a struggle with shift work, usually because their social activities interfere with getting adequate sleep between shifts!

Jetlag

Although this is very much like shift work, with disruption of the body clock, it has its own particular complications, such as: whether the flight is at night or during the day, the stress and strains of getting to and from as well as waiting at the airport, flight delays, arduous flights, sudden climate changes, etc. For example, flights from the UK to the USA mostly depart around midday and arrive about mid-afternoon local time, which is evening back at home. The afternoon bright light of the States, together with a cup or two of (caffeinated) coffee, can keep one going, hopefully until at least until 9 or 10pm local time, when bed might at last be contemplated. Nevertheless, the subsequent waking up in the small hours of the local US morning is aggravating to say the least. Taking a sleeping tablet at this time is not advisable, because it would be the same as doing so at one's normal morning wake-up time back home, when fairly alert. So, a higher dose is needed to be effective, leading to unwanted grogginess a few hours later and, probably, it will worsen the jetlag. Another solution, given that it is still dark at this early hour in the USA, is that some people find a melatonin tablet to be helpful then (that is, at 3–4am local time)—to trick the body clock into extending its night—but one should avoid all but dim indoor light until the desired getting up time. During the following day (US local time), a short (10 minute) nap will help, together with more caffeine—above all, seek plenty of daylight, especially just before the local dusk. Keep going until well into the evening, with the aid of bright indoor lighting. If a melatonin tablet is to be contemplated once more, then do not take at bedtime, but, as before, on waking up later, in the early hours. This regimen should hasten adaptation to US time.

Eastbound travel is more difficult for the body clock to cope with and adapt to because the day is shortened. This can be further complicated in the case of flying from the USA to the UK, because these flights are mostly overnight, with a bleary-eyed arrival into the British morning, and maybe having had little sleep on the flight. If the body clock was already set to US time, then the best way for a quicker adaptation is not to crash out in bed for a full sleep, soon after arrival. Instead, take no more than a couple of hours of sleep that morning (a short nap is not sufficient if there has been little sleep on the plane), and then seek plenty of daylight, some caffeine, and keep going until the evening—maybe hang on until 10pm (UK time). There will be little problem sleeping then, of course, because of the previously poor sleep on the plane. Now, however, the difficulty is waking up next morning, when the body clock thinks that it is in the middle of the night, as in the USA. After struggling out of bed, and watching everyone else tucking into their breakfast, go for more daylight and caffeine!

For those relying on a melatonin tablet, and having gone eastbound, it should not be taken on waking up on the next morning as was the case for westbound travel. Instead, take it early evening, about a few hours before the intended bedtime. This helps convince the body clock that it is indeed night-time rather than afternoon as it was in the USA. Evening bright light should be avoided after taking this tablet—and no caffeine either! A few more nights like this, with an early evening melatonin tablet, dim light in the evening but bright light on struggling out of bed the next morning, should speed up adaptation to UK time. A word of caution—melatonin tablets do not work for everyone, and the advice I have given is only advice, not advocacy!

Successful adaptation to a new time zone not only depends on the extent of the time change, eastbound versus westbound travel, but, also, natural differences between people. Again, 'owls' seem to cope quicker with jetlag than 'larks', but there are other unknown reasons that may well be in one's genes. Roughly speaking, for westbound travel, and without the aid of melatonin tablets, it takes about a day and night (that is, 24 hours) for every hour of time-zone shift, for at least some adaptation to set in. For example, about five days will be needed to become fairly accustomed to New York time, having arrived from the UK. As it takes longer to adapt to eastbound travel, then allow roughly about three days and nights of adaptation for every two hours of time-zone shift—that is, about a week to shift five hours having come from New York to the UK. Of course, judicious use of local daylight, as appropriate, could well speed all this up.

Good night

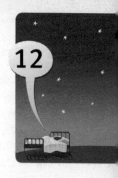

Self-reports

The simplest way of measuring sleep is to ask people to keep a 'sleep diary', and write down each night when they go to bed, switch off the light, etc. Next morning they note when they wake up and get out of bed and, on a rating scale, how well they slept, for example: extremely well, very well, cannot say, rather badly, very badly. Sometimes it is best to remove 'cannot say' and substitute a term such as 'fairly well', to encourage people to make a more definite decision. Also, we could ask whether they woke up in the night, what caused it, and whether they can remember for how long they were awake. All this is very subjective, of course, and can contain many inaccuracies and omissions. However it is easy to gather such information.

With my colleagues, Dr Louise Reyner and Francesca Pankhurst, a few years ago we undertook a very large study of sleep disturbance[1] in 400 people (211 women and 189 men) aged between 20 and 70 years, who were recruited one per household. Eight locations in England were used, with 50 recruits from each. As they had to be sleeping in their homes at night, we had to exclude those doing night work, as well as those suffering from physical illnesses and pain that seriously disrupted sleep. Also, as we wanted to study fairly normal sleepers, we excluded those taking sleeping tablets and other medications taken to aid sleep (including alcohol), but we did include all other 'poor sleepers'. About one in twenty volunteers fell into these latter categories and had to be excluded. Everyone kept a sleep diary for 15 consecutive nights, including the two weekends. Men and women were divided into three age groups: 20–34 years (80 women and 68 men), 35–49 years (73 women and 62 men), and 50–70 years (58 women and

59 men). Thus, the study was fairly representative of the adult population and was one of the largest of its sort ever undertaken in the UK. As it provides useful information about people's typical sleep habits, I will describe some of the more interesting findings.

On some nights the participants forgot to complete their logs, but out of the possible total of 6,000 nights we obtained information on 5,718 (95.3 per cent) of them. I should add that people were paid a modest amount per night to participate. Figure 6 shows the go-to-bed time reported for these 5,718 nights, when the most likely time was between 11pm and midnight, although women went to bed somewhat earlier than men. As might be expected, fewer people go to bed after midnight and before 11pm.

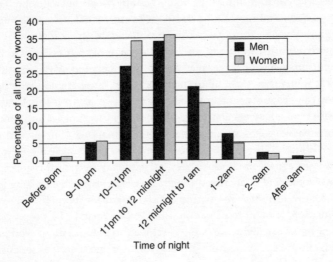

Time of night

Figure 6 Going to bed.

Estimates of the time taken to go to sleep, from 'lights out', are shown in Figure 7, where it can be seen that for most nights this period was between 10 and 30 minutes, although, for around a quarter of the nights, it was well beyond this. Men and women under 50 years of age did not differ much in this respect, but for the 50 to 70 year olds, men reported falling asleep faster, averaging 13 minutes

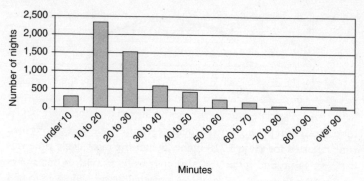

Figure 7 Time taken to go to sleep.

compared with 22 minutes for the women. Older women do commonly report more difficulty in getting to sleep.

Most people finally woke up between 6 and 8am, with women waking up somewhat later, by something like 20 minutes, as can be seen from Figure 8. Remember, these findings included weekend lie-ins as well. From the individual 'going to sleep' and 'final waking up' reports we were also able to calculate, for every hour of the night, the percentages of people who were asleep. Figure 9 includes those people who may have woken up for a while during the night but wanted to

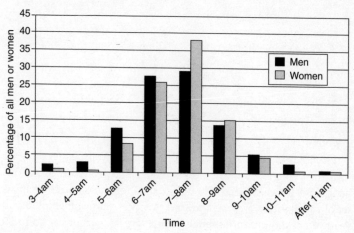

Figure 8 Wake-up time.

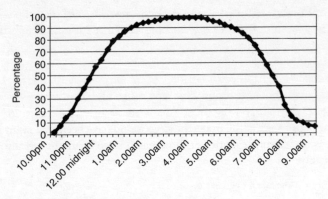

Figure 9 Percentage of people asleep over the night.

return to sleep. On no occasion over the night was everyone asleep, but between 3 and 5am it was close, at 98 per cent.

One of the most important findings was the amount of sleep recorded in these logs, and I will reveal this later (see Chapter 18) when I come to this fairly hot topic. I will also look at what caused them to wake in the night. Meanwhile, here is how they rated the quality of their sleep the following morning. Figure 10 is based on

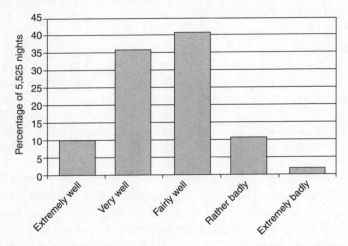

Figure 10 'Last night I slept . . .'.

5,525 nights, slightly fewer than before, because they sometimes forgot to fill in this part of the morning sleep log. For most nights they slept well, although, for one in eight nights, sleep was rated more on the bad side.

A good night's sleep is one that is uninterrupted, with few awakenings, and should leave us feeling refreshed and alert during the day except, perhaps, for the natural dip in the early afternoon—although the bigger the dip the worse the sleep would have been that night. So, it is not simply a matter of 'how much sleep' at night but also its quality.

Moving

The saying, to 'sleep like a top', was first used around 400 years ago, and is still synonymous with sound sleep. The 'top' was a child's spinning top, which remains quite still when spinning. Indeed, the antithesis of both stillness and good sleep is excessive movement, and is why the measurement of body movement during sleep is a fairly good, simple index of sleep quality. As movement increases beyond the normal levels, people will increasingly find that their sleep was not so good, although they may not realise how disturbed it was. For this reason people's perceptions of their sleep, as in the sleep diaries that I have just described, are not particularly reliable when it comes to sleep quality, and I must turn to more 'objective measures'. Let me start with body movement. When we move in bed, almost invariably so does at least one arm—which makes the wrist a particularly convenient place to place a movement sensor. This is done with a small, almost unnoticeable, wrist-worn device called an 'actimeter' (as in the Actiwatch®, for example[2]), the size of a small wristwatch, which contains a movement detector and memory chip that stores the number of movements every few seconds throughout sleep. Data are downloaded into a computer and the printout is an 'actigram'.

Our 400 participants wore actimeters every night; at least they were supposed to, but occasionally they forgot to put theirs on. Fortunately, we lost only 4 per cent in this way, leaving 5,742 nights that were OK. People normally wake up momentarily about four to six times per hour, just to turn over and get more comfortable, and as

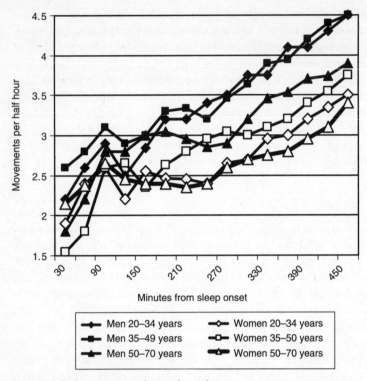

Figure 11 Body movements during the night.

these arousals are so short they are of no consequence. There are fewer movements at the beginning of sleep, because it is deeper, but these gradually increase as sleep becomes lighter throughout the night. Figure 11 shows the average movement for every 30 minutes over the night for all the nights, divided up into the three age groups, for both men and women. Although all six groups show the overall trend of increasing movements as sleep progressed, two features are very clear: first, for each age group men move around more than women and, second, both older men and older women move less than their younger counterparts.

Frequent brief arousals, not just to turn over, but lasting many seconds, indicate more serious sleep disturbance, and may be the result of 'sleep apnoea' or 'periodic leg movements', described in detail in Chapter 21. To know that we have woken up during sleep, we usually have to be awake for at least a minute or so, otherwise there is no recollection of it next morning. This is why sufferers with numerous very short awakenings, maybe lasting only 10–15 seconds at a time, have no idea that their sleep is so bad and are puzzled as to why they are so sleepy in the daytime.

13 Brain waves

Ripples and rollers

We can feign sleep by lying still for several minutes but remaining awake with closed eyes, and even fool the actimeter into registering that we are asleep. Fortunately, there is more to sleep than an absence of body movement, and better ways of measuring sleep are available. Sleep is not only mainly for our cortex; of all the body's organs, it is the brain, and especially the cortex, that show the clearest and most profound changes during sleep. That something special happens to the cortex in sleep ties in with the most obvious effect of sleep loss—sleepiness—which, of course, is caused by the brain. Changes shown by most, if not all, other body organs in sleep are just as likely to be seen in relaxed wakefulness and not exclusive to sleep.

Not surprisingly, the brain shows clear sleep-related changes that cannot be feigned. These can be seen in the EEG (electroencephalogram—'brain waves'). The EEG is detected using tiny (one centimetre in diameter) silver discs ('electrodes') glued to the scalp through the parted hair. Being sited directly above the cortex, they pick up brain waves largely from the cortex, rather than from deeper inside the brain, which is very convenient for us, because this is precisely the part of the brain in which we are interested, anyway. Easier said than done, however, because these brain waves are so small that to measure them they have to be amplified a millionfold, using sophisticated equipment. Like waves in the water, these waves alter in height and in number, from little ripples to big rollers, as consciousness changes from alert wakefulness (for example, when we are looking around), to drowsiness, and then to sleep.

Whereas much of sleep can be assessed from the EEG alone, dreaming sleep, otherwise known as REM sleep, because of its characteristic and eponymous rapid eye movements, is a rather peculiar form of sleep because its EEG is like that of drowsiness or light 'non-REM' sleep. In contrast, for many other mammals the EEG of REM sleep is more like that of alert wakefulness, and for this reason REM sleep has also been called 'paradoxical' sleep—that is, the animal is clearly asleep, but the EEG indicates that it is awake and hence the paradox! To clarify matters, we also measure the rapid eye movements as well, and just to make absolutely sure that this is REM sleep, and that the sleeper is somehow not simulating these rapid eye movements, there is another, final, fail-safe measure for REM sleep. For some peculiar reason, tension in the muscles around the chin and jaws almost disappears during REM sleep, but not during the rest of (non-REM) sleep, and cannot be feigned during wakefulness.

Apart from the rapid eye movements of REM sleep, it is also useful to monitor eye movements when someone is falling asleep, more so when they are struggling to stay awake, because the eyelids slowly droop, then shut, and slowly open only to shut again, with the eyes rolling up and down in their sockets in the opposite direction. Hence, the term used for this is 'eye rolling'. It happens in those microsleeps mentioned in earlier chapters, except that with microsleeps the drowsy individual usually wakes up.

By using the EEG we can describe sleep in terms of 'light sleep' (small waves), 'deep sleep' (otherwise called 'slow-wave sleep', because of those large EEG waves), and REM sleep. Light and deep sleep are collectively called 'non-REM' sleep, which is a bit of an insult—describing the majority of sleep (light and deep sleep) by what it is not. As might be expected, it is much easier to wake someone up from light than from deep sleep, whereas REM sleep is odd in this respect because it is both light and deep—I explain this in Chapter 14.

Let me be a little more technical about the sleep EEG, but only for a moment. Both light and deep non-REM sleep can each be divided further, with light sleep into stages 1 and 2 and deep sleep into stages 3 and 4. Stage 1 is synonymous with 'drowsiness', and is usually short-lived because it is *en route* to stage 2, which is a prolific stage of sleep occupying around half of the night's sleep. Stage 2 contains two

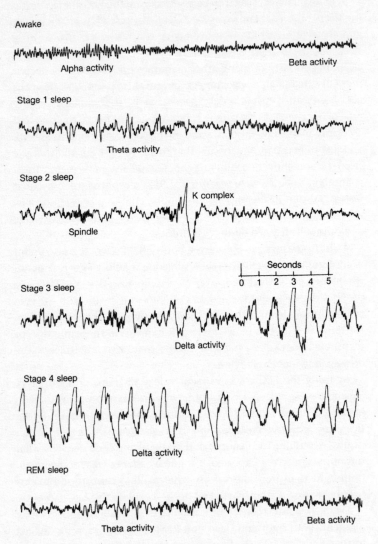

Figure 12 EEG characteristics of different sleep stages.

interesting EEG characteristics: occasional, single 'big rollers' (typical of deep sleep), called 'K complexes', and bursts of what are called 'sleep spindles'. Both K complexes and spindles are thought to help maintain sleep and block out harmless external noises and other potential disturbances to sleep. Illustrations of all these brain waves are seen in Figure 12, beginning with the awake EEG and its rather nondescript small ripples of beta activity, which are typical of alert wakefulness and found when we are looking around. This contrasts with the more distinctive, larger ripples of alpha activity, found during relaxed wakefulness, which are most apparent when the eyes are shut and there is nothing particular on one's mind. Drowsiness and stage 1 sleep are characterised by more distinct slower ripples, or theta waves, which are not as slow or as high as the rollers of deep sleep. A microsleep largely consists of theta waves. Stage 2 can be seen in Figure 12, with its characteristic spindle and K complex. As more and more K complexes appear and start to join together, this is called stage 3 sleep; this, in turn, gives way to virtually continuous K complexes that typify stage 4, producing an EEG full of these huge rolling waves.

Just to repeat, stage 3 and stage 4 sleep are together called 'deep sleep' or 'slow-wave sleep', which makes up about 10–20 per cent of a typical night's sleep in a young adult. REM sleep comprises another 20–25 per cent. About 5–10 per cent of sleep consists of brief awakenings and stage 1, which together with stage 2 comprises 'light sleep', makes up the other half of sleep. REM sleep appears about every 90 minutes throughout sleep, and in doing so breaks sleep up into characteristic 90-minute cycles. Deep sleep is usually loaded towards the first two to three cycles in the first half of sleep. To be more precise, deep sleep (especially stage 4) is most intense soon after sleep onset, with smaller reappearances thereafter. All this can be seen in the 'hypnogram' of the distribution of sleep stages and the cycling, in the typical young adult (Figure 13).

Let me now revert to the simpler terminology of the three types of sleep: light (that is, stages 1 and 2), deep (stages 3 and 4), and REM sleep. Besides, the division of non-REM sleep into stages 1–4 is rather arbitrary, albeit appealing, but I am not sure that it serves much purpose any more, other than as a useful illustration of how the sleep

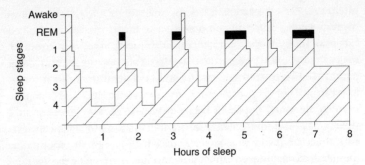

Figure 13 Hypnogram.

EEG changes over the night, and it may be clouding our real understanding of sleep.

Really slow waves

The amount of deep sleep depends on the length of previous wakefulness—the longer we are awake, the more the deep sleep, especially during the first one or two sleep cycles. For this reason, deep sleep seems to be the type of sleep that is most likely to be linked with cortical recovery, especially because deep sleep is most intense in the frontal cortex—the region of the cortex working particularly hard during wakefulness. It is often claimed that older adults have little by way of deep sleep, suggesting that somehow the older brain has 'seized up', although all that mostly happens is that, with ageing, the big rollers of deep sleep become shallower, more difficult to spot, and thinly spread out. But they are still there, albeit somewhat fewer in number.

In contrast, REM does not increase with increasing wakefulness, but becomes more prolific as sleep progresses, being most apparent towards the end of sleep. This is also seen in the hypnogram, with successive periods of REM sleep becoming longer—that is, REM sleep largely depends on how much sleep has preceded it. Suggesting that it is not particularly linked to recovery from wakefulness; more likely, it is linked to a recovery from sleep itself. More about this in Chapter 14, although suffice it to say that, if we assume that the need for sleep will decline as sleep progresses towards its natural end, the increasing appearance of REM sleep suggests that it is not so vital as is often assumed. I should add, however, that REM sleep is also influenced by the body clock, and part of the reason for its increase at the end of the night is the accompanying rise in body temperature, from its daily trough.

Deep sleep, unlike REM sleep, is hardly affected by the body clock—really only by the length of prior wakefulness—which probably holds the key to why we really need sleep, especially deep sleep. Inasmuch as deep sleep with its slow waves seems to reflect some sort of recovery for the cortex, deep sleep also contains some particularly slow waves, and it is probably not 'any old slow wave' that really counts, here, but those really slow ones that have a frequency of around 1 cycle/second. This is a fairly new discovery, and these very slow waves seem to be the ones that may well be linked to the 're-organisation of plastic circuits within the cortex' during sleep, and more closely linked to the workload of the waking cortex. Moreover, these very slow waves are most evident in the frontal cortex, and we owe much of this new insight to the pioneering work of the late Professor Merica Steriade, in Quebec.[1] This is a tantalising area of research, as my colleague Dr Clare Anderson and I have found out.[2]

Brain work

It is generally thought that our need for sleep (especially these particularly slow waves), accumulates during wakefulness in a way that is not really affected by what we do when awake—whether this is lying relaxed without a care in the world, watching an exciting ball game or movie, or even studying hard for an exam. Even physical exercise, such as a moderate workout in the gym, or a cool jog on a familiar course with eyes down or just staring ahead, will not affect that night's sleep, largely because the body and its muscles can adequately recover afterwards during wakefulness. The relaxation and peace of mind that come from a satisfying jog in the early evening might well make a poor sleeper sleep better, but this is more of a psychological effect.

There is something else, quite intriguing, however, that seems to depend on whether or not one becomes particularly hot during the exercise. If one does, the subsequent sleep is deeper—with even more slow waves, although I must add that these slow waves are more of the 'general sort' and not necessarily the very slow waves, because the work I am about to describe happened before interest turned towards those very slow waves. Returning to exercise and sleep, and contrary to what I have said, this might indicate that muscles need sleep after all—when pushed to their limits. I spent some years trying to unravel this effect, and it seems that critical to all this is simply how hot we become, irrespective of the exercise. More to the point, it is how hot the brain becomes, because a hot body also means a hot brain, with a speeding up of all the brain's activities, especially those of the cortex, making it work harder. Accordingly, more cortical recovery is needed during sleep, reflected by more deep sleep.

More clues came from our findings that identical amounts of very heavy exercise in a cold wind, to stop the body heating up, have no effect on sleep. Another, most enjoyable experiment for all concerned was just to let volunteers lie in a warm bath—no exercise whatsoever, to heat up gently, to the same extent as in heavy exercise. Again, this resulted in more slow waves that night. Now, it could be argued that perhaps muscle warmth is still behind all this, and that is where our final experiment came in. To some extent the brain can be heated up a little, on its own, and initially with much less effect on the rest of the body, by blowing warm air on to the cheeks and face. Remember, in Chapter 6 I mentioned 'flushing cheeks' and how these help keep the brain cool; well, the reverse can be done with warm air blown on to the waking face with the outcome being more slow waves that night!

Finally, and to return to the topic of sleep providing muscles with little or no extra benefit beyond physical rest for their recovery after exercise, many studies including our own have looked at the effects of sleep loss on the ability to run or cycle. Even five days without any sleep whatsoever has no effect on the physical capacity to do this, which would otherwise be expected if sleep provided some unique benefits, here. Although sleepiness makes us less inclined to do exercise, the failing is with psychological rather than physical stamina.

Even for the most idle but alert waking person, the cortex will be busy, waiting for action, and in that 'quiet readiness'. It becomes even busier when bombarded with lots of new and interesting information coming in from the senses, especially from the eyes, because vision is our most important sense in dealing with more information from the outside world. In fact, of all the senses put together (that is, hearing, touch, taste, smell, and balance, as well as sight) more than a third of all the input into the brain comes from the eyes. Nevertheless, real 'brain (cortical) strain' comes not from passively watching the TV or looking at a colourful magazine, or sitting an exam, but from walking within a richly varied environment, taking in all the information from the senses (especially vision), and 'making sense' of it all. Window shopping, sightseeing, and visiting a museum or gallery are good examples, as is, for that matter, anything new, fascinating and absorbing, especially if it is sustained for a few hours. The eventual feeling of weariness and, I suspect, the accompanying aching feet, are not the result of excessive walking but a subtle cry from the brain to reduce this bombardment and just sit down and stop, because it cannot take any more!

'Getting out and about' like this not only provides healthy exercise for the body, muscles, lungs, and heart, but also exercises the cortex, because this rich sensory stimulation, far more than when sitting indoors, keeps the cortex in trim. The idea that regular brisk walking keeps the brain 'well oxygenated' and that any improvement in mental ability in older people is simply the result of the exercise overlooks this other benefit to the cortex, which must be better than simply pedalling on a monotonous exercise bicycle and staring at a wall, or running in a semi-trance while jogging outdoors. This, I believe, is critical to the concept of 'use it or lose it' in relation to daily mental activity and the subsequent need for sleep—and moreover, to what underlies the need for those very slow waves that help keep the cortex 'plastic, flexible, and adaptable'.

We take for granted our extraordinarily complex vision, with its superb facility to see colour, excellent visual acuity, and capacity to see depth. Then there is the refined ability to move our eyes to scan a scene, as well as our remarkable skills in eye–hand co-ordination. No other mammal has this level of visual sophistication, which means that our ability to appreciate the visual environment is ideally suited to scenes rich in colour, detail, depth, movement, and panorama. Remember, we are naturally very curious animals, much more so than other adult mammals—a continually changing environment maintains our interest and heightened awareness and, of course, keeps the cortex on its toes. For many other mammals, smell is their dominant sense, or maybe hearing, and these are the senses that dominate their brains. A stimulating and engrossing environment for the rat and its acute sense of smell is a garbage tip at night, which for us is dull, almost invisible, and offensive!

Not only does a busy day sightseeing, window shopping, and visiting a museum bring on aching feet but also, often, a desire for an 'early night' after such an exhausting day. It may also be why we sleep so well on holiday—after all that new stimulation. Of course, other reasons, apart from the 'ozone' and 'sea air', may well be those evening sundowners at the bar, and getting away from the pressures of home and work. Nevertheless, when I studied this in a systematic way, by sending people off on a supervised sightseeing tour when they expected to spend the day in the dull laboratory, not only were they more sleepy in the evening, but their sleep was deeper with more slow waves. Another group of less lucky people had an unexpected few hours just walking round a large but dull hall, to replicate the walking endured by the sightseers. No changes, here, with evening sleepiness, sleep or slow waves, and interestingly no aching feet!

Incredibly dull studies, not by me I should add, asking volunteers to spend most of the waking day with the eyes shut or staring at a blank wall do not change sleep or lead to fewer slow waves during deep sleep. Nor does spending several days lying on a bed, wearing translucent goggles, getting up only to eat and go to the toilet. Not surprisingly, much of the time in this latter experiment was spent dozing or asleep, with lots more REM and light sleep. Even in wakefulness under these dreary conditions, the cortex still remains in its 'quiet readiness'—ready and probably hoping for some action. To these ends it still needs its deep sleep, because the lack of daytime stimulation does not point to a lesser need for this.

REM sleep

14

Jerky eyes

The link between eye movements and dreaming was first suggested a long time ago, with one of the earliest accounts appearing in 1892, from a Professor G.T. Ladd, a professor of mental and moral philosophy at Yale University. He reported, through pure introspection about his own sleep, that during deep dreamless sleep his eyes were stationary, but during dreaming sleep he was 'inclined also to believe that, in somewhat vivid visual dreams, the eyeballs move gently in their sockets, taking various positions . . .'.[1] How he came up with this idea is a mystery because neither Ladd nor his associates actually watched the eyes of sleepers. This would have been a simple task because the rapid eye movements of REM sleep can easily be seen under the eyelids. Such observations were not made until 1930, when Dr E. Jacobson, having noticed that when waking people move their eyes on trying to recollect some visual event, also saw these eye movements in sleep, during what appeared to be dreaming. Later, in his popular book, *You Can Sleep Well—the ABC's of restful sleep for the average person*, published in 1938, he suggested 'watch the sleeper whose eyes move under his closed lids . . . awaken him . . . you are likely to find that . . . he had seen something in a dream'.[2]

It took another 17 years for this connection to be made properly, in 1955, by Eugene Aserinsky (with Nathaniel Kleitman), at the University of Chicago, who first referred to these eye movements within REM sleep as 'jerky eye movements', but soon renamed them as rapid eye movements—and changed the name of dreaming sleep to REM sleep. Although dreaming is most vivid and intense during REM sleep, milder, more reflective, and less fantastic forms of dreaming occur throughout much of the rest of (non-REM) sleep. Moreover, we do not always dream during REM sleep, as these Chicago investigators had also noted that, out of 27 awakenings of sleepers showing rapid eye movements, on only 20 occasions were there accounts of dreaming with visual imagery.

Without doubt REM sleep is the most fascinating form of sleep, and it is not surprising that so much of sleep research has been directed towards it. There certainly is much more to REM sleep than meets the eye, even though most of it contains no eye movements at all, because they appear only in periodic bursts, occupying a minority of REM sleep. Besides, they have nothing to do with the dream imagery itself, as dreaming is probably just a later add-on to REM sleep. Dreams are created in the cortex, whereas REM sleep is produced deep within the brain by regions that cannot themselves dream. If the cortex is destroyed, REM sleep simply carries on without the dreaming, but the penile erections continue in the male, which are another curious phenomenon of REM sleep. REM sleep appears early in our development, even in the fetus and, as I have already mentioned, it is quite distinct from the rest of sleep. In fact, it is more like wakefulness, which is the starting point for my argument that maybe we should view REM sleep not as 'true sleep' but as a type of wakefulness, or rather 'non-wakefulness'—rather like the 'screen-saver' mode on a computer.

Confinement

In the month or so before birth we have more REM sleep than at any other time of our lives, when it occupies more than half of sleep, at around 8–10 hours per day. This contrasts with the nightly 100 minutes or so, for the adult. All this can be seen in Figure 14, where REM sleep declines rapidly after birth to about five hours a day by the end of the first year. This plunge also argues against the idea that REM sleep is critical for processing memories, because it cannot explain why, when the baby's brain is so bombarded with new experiences and learning, so much of REM sleep disappears. By the way, such a loss is not compensated by any increase in the intensity of REM sleep.

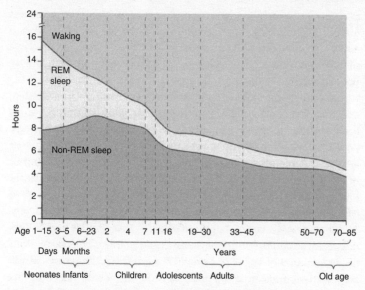

Figure 14 Daily sleep during our lifespan. (From Roffwarg *et al.*[3])

Instead, the most plausible reason for this drop in REM sleep is the theory[3] that it provides the pre-birth brain with much needed stimulation to allow it to develop properly—a level of stimulation that it would not otherwise get within the muffled and dark confines of the uterus. Thus, REM sleep provides substitute stimulation for the brain, by generating 'pseudo-stimulation' from within the brain itself. When the baby is born it has real stimulation from the outside world and, as there is no substitute for the real world, REM sleep diminishes. Nevertheless, some REM sleep remains with us throughout life, probably keeping the cortex periodically stimulated and 'tweaked up' during sleep, in the absence of wakefulness, because the cortex dislikes long periods of inactivity. Moreover, without this periodic stimulation from REM sleep, we might not be able to detect danger or predators so effectively, and would otherwise be particularly groggy and confused if suddenly woken up, and less able to respond to danger.

Fragile

Rapid eye movement sleep can be a very fragile state, as a restless night's sleep is usually at the expense of REM sleep—which is why poor sleepers are more likely to remember their dreams, because it is the accompanying REM sleep from which they usually wake, unlike the good sleeper who is oblivious to all. It is fragile because the brain is not really unconscious during REM sleep, because we seem to be fairly vigilant to what is going on around us. Whispering a familiar name or providing some other meaningful sound to someone slumbering in REM sleep will usually produce an instant awakening, whereas a fairly loud and meaningless noise, even a train thundering past (if you live beside a railway), will be ignored, provided that it is not annoying. Annoyance or the emotional significance of the sound is particularly important in determining whether we wake up from REM sleep. Even in our enlightened age of the equality of the sexes, the crying baby is more likely to wake up mum than dad, and from REM sleep. Whereas the neighbour's barking dog will probably wake up both of them from REM sleep, the overflying aircraft may well wake up only dad who gets particularly annoyed by these aircraft, but not mum, who may have other matters to worry about. Infants, by the way, usually sleep well—it takes a lot of noise to wake them up, unlike more meaningful hunger and a filled nappy. These examples of vigilance during REM sleep contrast with our poor state of awareness during deep non-REM sleep, when we are truly out for the count, and where it is more a matter of the loudness of a sound, rather than its meaning, that will eventually wake us up.

More or less

Almost all mammals have REM sleep, except for those dolphins and seals at sea mentioned in Chapter 1, where REM sleep is absent. This may also be the case for other members of the whale family. Who knows whether or how these marine animals dream? Given that many of them sleep with one side of the brain at a time, it certainly would be strange, if not bizarre, to have one side awake and the other dreaming—how would they know what is fact and what is fantasy given that there are predators around? Best not to have any dreams at all perhaps. We humans can also lose all our REM sleep, for weeks, months, or even a year at a time, through what seems to be a harmless side effect of some common and effective medicines for treating depression, which have been taken by millions of patients world wide. The contribution (if any) that this absence of REM sleep makes to the treatment of depression is unclear, especially as improvement of the depression is not evident until after several weeks of treatment, whereas the suppression of REM sleep by these medicines is immediate.

When antidepressant treatment is stopped there is some rebound increase of REM sleep, but this amounts to only a fraction of what has been lost—indicating no great pressure for us to have REM sleep. A heretical statement, perhaps, but let me continue this line of thinking. Maybe the periodic appearance of REM sleep during normal sleep is not the result of a build-up of REM sleep 'pressure' every 90 minutes, but is perhaps caused by the periodic cessation of non-REM sleep—that is, perhaps the remainder of sleep cannot be sustained continuously throughout sleep, and even it must rest up periodically? So, rather than us having to keep waking up every 90 minutes or so, REM sleep kicks in as a 'fall-back state' or allows the brain to go into 'screen-saver mode', allowing slumber to continue uninterrupted.

Healthy people who normally sleep for what seems to them an adequate seven or eight hours per night can easily extend their sleep for a few more hours if they so wish (see Chapter 18). This extra sleep is similar to that found in the last part of normal sleep, although it usually contains even more REM sleep, and can easily include over an hour of extra REM sleep. Despite this excess of REM sleep, the next night's sleep shows no similar REM sleep reduction. Interestingly, if the sleeper is prevented from having REM sleep during this extended sleep, by being woken up whenever it appears, there is still no change to the next night's REM sleep—all of which points to this extra REM sleep being superfluous. However, not all of REM sleep is so easily dispensable, because REM sleep during the first few hours of normal sleep is rather more robust, albeit still able to be suppressed by those antidepressants.

If essential brain recovery were proceeding during REM sleep, then it would be surprising how rapidly the brain could switch from REM sleep to alert wakefulness when we are suddenly woken up from it. There is little of the befuddlement that happens after awakening from deep sleep. This rapid switching from REM sleep to wakefulness points to REM sleep being particularly close to wakefulness—and that is the theme of Chapter 15.

Safety

Whether or not REM sleep is found in reptiles is a matter for debate, largely because their brains are so different from ours and because they are 'cold blooded'—all in all, it would be difficult to spot this type of sleep anyway. Undisputed REM sleep is certainly found in mammals and birds, although birds do not have much, because it comprises only about five per cent of their sleep. The two living, primitive egg-laying mammals (both found in Australia) seem to have huge amounts of what appears to be more primitive types of REM sleep and, in the case of the 'duckbilled platypus', this is around eight hours per day.[4]

For more typical mammals, safety when sleeping is the major influence on how much REM sleep they have—the more dangerous their sleeping arrangements, the less the REM sleep. For example, sheep and antelope have relatively little REM sleep, whereas the ferret has huge amounts and, in the adult animal, which sleeps for about 18 hours a day, 8 hours of this can be REM sleep. What is more, its REM sleep becomes more apparent as sleep progresses—just like us.

Within sleep, the extent of the cycling of REM sleep largely depends on brain size. Whereas for us adults it appears every 90 minutes, in babies it is 60 minutes and, in the adult rat, cat, and elephant, it is about 12, 30, and 120 minutes, respectively.

Paralysis

Another extraordinary happening during REM sleep is that we are paralysed, to prevent us from acting out our dreams; this paralysis is called 'atonia' (from the Latin 'without movement'). It is not the same as the profound relaxation that is seen in the jaw muscles, mentioned earlier, but something else. When we begin to fall asleep, the muscles that maintain body posture (in the back, trunk, neck, and limbs) become relaxed and go somewhat limp, with the most apparent effect being the head nodding forwards. This is not the atonia, however, which is special to REM sleep. Atonia can be likened to a car with the engine on, but unable to move because it is not in gear. No matter how much the driver decides to push the accelerator, nothing happens—the car is paralysed. Apart from the rapid eye movements of REM sleep, no other muscles over which we usually have control can be moved. Arms, legs, fingers, toes, and trunk are all paralysed. However, the muscles of the heart and other vital organs, over which we have no real control, continue to function normally. The tension in those paralysed muscles is similar to that of relaxed wakefulness—the activity within the muscles continues to tick over as normal—it is just that they cannot contract or move.

The atonia of REM sleep is produced by a small region that is deep down in the brain, called the 'locus ceruleus', which switches the paralysis on and off as soon as REM sleep begins and ends, respectively. Sometimes, the atonia continues momentarily into wakefulness, which is more likely if we are awoken suddenly and dramatically from REM sleep—from a nightmare, for example. It can be a frightening experience, because all that can be moved is the eyes, although this does not usually last for more than a minute. Moving the eyes very rapidly, if in this unfortunate state, can break the paralysis, as can being touched by someone. The problem is how will a bed partner recognise what is happening, because the jaws and mouth are also paralysed and we cannot speak or cry out? It is called 'sleep paralysis' and in this limited form usually nothing to worry about.

Pioneering studies on cats, by Professor Michel Jouvet in Lyons and Dr Adrian Morrison in Philadelphia, have shown that if the locus ceruleus is destroyed, to eliminate the atonia of REM sleep, then, when this sleep appears, the cat typically opens its eyes, stares, raises its head, searches, reaches and grasps, and may even stalk imaginary prey—seemingly acting out a dream. Its eyes are unseeing, because objects placed in front are ignored. Similarly, it will groom, but a piece of fluff placed on its fur will go unnoticed. Although sexual and feeding activities have never been seen in the cat in this state, there is often aggression and attacking behaviour, with hissing, pawing, raised hackles, and an arched back. All this seems to be 'play acting', albeit in a convincingly dramatic way, because the cat's real emotions seem to be switched off at this time. This might explain why the animal seldom wakes itself up from this bizarre, non-paralysed, REM sleep, given that REM sleep is a potentially fragile type of sleep. On the other hand, it will instantly wake up to a meaningful sound, such as the rattling of its food bowl. Such dream episodes last for about five minutes, and are usually followed by a brief awakening and the cat settling down to return to sleep.

Back to humans and the fragility of REM sleep. Whereas emotive external sounds will quickly awaken us from REM sleep, how is it that dreams, with all their emotional content, do not normally wake us up, except for the more frightening nightmares? Not only for the cat but for us as well, the dreamer seems to be emotionally 'numbed' and protected from the emotional content of the dream. This is also shown by the little or no increase in heart and breathing rates or in blood pressure (although these do become more irregular) during REM sleep, which would normally happen in wakefulness if we become excited in any way. Moreover, during REM sleep, blood levels of the 'fight or flight' and stress hormones, adrenaline (epinephrine) and cortisol, remain unchanged.

How all this emotional blocking is achieved is not clear, although important regions of the brain that control emotional behaviour, such as the 'amygdala', are very active in REM sleep, which may in part be the result of their blocking these emotions. The amygdala is probably the 'guardian of REM sleep', because here is where the sleeping brain's main 'watchkeeper' resides, somehow keeping us vigilant to external threats. In wakefulness, this part of the brain helps us to assess dangerous situations, respond to threats, decide when these are likely to occur, and even create the feeling of fear. Damage to the amygdala causes us to become less fearful, not to recognise danger so easily, and to fail to recognise many emotions in other people.

By the way, 'REM sleep without atonia' is not the 'sleepwalking' that typically occurs in deep non-REM sleep (see Chapter 22). Obviously, the usual paralysis of REM sleep would prevent sleepwalking, anyway. Nevertheless, some people, usually healthy adult men, can show something similar to those cats, which is called 'REM sleep behaviour disorder' (RBD). Sufferers usually have REM sleep with the normal paralysis but, for unknown reasons, the paralysis occasionally lifts during REM sleep, when the accompanying dreams are often different from normal, in being much more aggressive, confrontational, and violent (but apparently not sexual). Needless to say, bed partners can be at risk during these episodes.

Whereas we can shiver in non-REM sleep, the paralysis of REM sleep also means that we cannot do this to warm up, if we happen to be cold during REM sleep. This may seem unimportant, because all we have to do is pull up the duvet. It is more interesting, however, that other ways in which our body temperature is controlled are also impaired during REM sleep, and not as a result of the paralysis. For example, if we become too hot during REM sleep, we cannot sweat very easily, but can do so in non-REM sleep. All of this is rather like the state of affairs found in normal healthy waking babies, whether they are awake or asleep, because they cannot shiver or sweat at all—both of which come with later development. Babies are quite safe, however, because nature has provided a back-up system. If they get cold, instead of shivering, they can generate more body heat by 'burning up' a special form of fat, called 'brown fat', located in large amounts between their shoulders and near the heart. It is like turning on an immersion heater, and is the reason why babies will not get so cold as parents might think. Most adults still have some brown fat (elsewhere in the body), but not as much as in the baby. The reason for my digression to waking babies is that adult temperature regulation in REM sleep is rather like that of the baby, whether awake or asleep. Although we adults cannot shiver during REM sleep we can still 'burn' this brown fat. This, together with the other peculiarities of body temperature control during REM sleep, points to REM sleep regressing to an earlier level of our development, unlike non-REM sleep, which is more 'advanced'. More about this later.

Bursts of activity

The rapid eye movements of REM sleep are usually side-to-side ('saccadic') movements, just like those in wakefulness, as if we were scanning a new scene, but these particular eye movements have nothing to do with the dream imagery. Typically, they appear in bursts lasting about 20 seconds, followed by a longer period of quiescence, although they do become more intense as the night progresses. The latter indicates a sleep sufficiency, because the bursts reach a peak of intensity after about seven hours of sleep, and are least intense at the beginning of the night.

Accompanying each burst of rapid eye movements is an intriguing electrical activity initiated from deep below the cortex, called 'PGO waves' (from three brain areas—the pons, geniculate thalamus, and occiput areas). They vary in intensity just as the eye movement bursts do, and both are also accompanied by small, almost unnoticeable twitches of the fingers and toes. These waves are largely absent from the rest of (non-REM) sleep, but something very similar occurs in wakefulness whenever an animal is alerted to a new stimulus, when it will prick up its ears and look towards whatever is causing the interest. In humans, however, these waves are difficult to detect without the aid of electrodes deeply implanted in the brain. In REM sleep, PGO waves are not usually in response to some external stimulation, such as noise, but are spontaneous, unlike those in wakefulness. Nevertheless, they still bombard the cortex as if it were being stimulated externally. It is as if, in the absence of its usual bombardment by the waking senses, the sleeping cortex needs to be stimulated periodically, which is what PGO waves may be doing. I mentioned at the start of this chapter that the developing cortex, within the confines of the mother's uterus, is in need of intense stimulation and it is the PGO waves in REM sleep that probably provide this. Something similar continues to happen during our adult REM sleep, except that in the baby this stimulation is more intense.

During the ongoing PGO bombardment in REM sleep, our cortex probably tries to make some sense of all these weird pseudo-sensations, by creating imagined events around them through dreaming. The disjointed nature of dreams, leaping from one unexpected theme to another, reflects this. Not all the cortex is involved in dreaming, however, because the frontal cortex, which in wakefulness helps us sustain attention to a particular event and ignore distractions, either cannot cope with all this distraction during REM sleep and shuts down, or purposely switches off so that it can continue to rest and recover. For whatever reason, it means that the rest of the cortex is freed from the frontal region's usual constraints, to go off and play, so to speak—hence, the unfettered distractions and leaps of imagination within dreams that make them so unpredictable, incoherent, and fascinating.

I mentioned that the intensity of the rapid eye movements (and PGO waves) within successive periods of REM sleep increase as sleep progresses. It is as if we need more and more of this internal distraction, either to maintain sleep and delay waking, or to prepare the brain for the waking day—or both. What is more, the novelty and unexpectedness of dreams distract the sleeper from being awoken by insignificant, meaningless noises and other stimuli from the outside world—which helps counteract the fragility of this sleep and the propensity to wake up, even though the brain's sentinel (the amygdala) maintains a 'watchful eye', for danger. Similarly, when awake, we can be absorbed by a TV programme and ignore trivial distractions while subconsciously remaining aware of what else is going on, and respond if needed. In many respects, REM sleep and dreaming are similar to this scenario.

Primitive?

Whereas non-REM sleep is largely a product of the more advanced parts of the brain, especially the cortex, REM sleep, on the other hand, originates from deep down in those areas of the brain looking after more basic brain and body functions. In this sense, and again, REM sleep can be seen to be rather 'primitive'. Moreover, if the cortex is removed, the animal will continue to show REM sleep but little of what we know to be non-REM sleep. The continued presence of REM sleep in the absence of a cortex suggests that it has other, more basic functions than just keeping the cortex periodically stimulated during sleep. These 'primitive' brain areas also affect our general level of arousal whether we are awake or asleep, to the extent that REM sleep seems to be on a different dimension to that of non-REM sleep. In pursuing this idea I argue in the next Chapter that REM sleep is not 'true sleep', as is non-REM sleep, but a more primitive state wherein wake-fulness is turned off rather than sleep turned on.

15 Or REM wakefulness?

Screen saver

Earlier, I mentioned that the similarity between rapid eye movement (REM) sleep and wakefulness is the reason why, for most other mammals, REM sleep is also called 'paradoxical' sleep. Whereas the EEG of human REM sleep is slightly different, being more like that of very light sleep, in both humans and other mammals there are striking similarities between REM sleep and wakefulness. For example, other types of EEG activity in the brain, called 'gamma' and 'hippocampal theta' waves, normally found in alert wakefulness, are also to be seen in REM sleep, but not in the remainder of (non-REM) sleep. Hippocampal theta appears when an animal intends to move, and gamma activity indicates that different parts of the cortex are co-ordinating themselves for action.

Staying technical for a few moments more, certain of the brain's chemical neurotransmitters, acetylcholine and a substance called gamma-aminobutyric acid (or GABA for short), show similar changes in both REM sleep and wakefulness, which are different from those of the rest of sleep. But it has to be said that, although many aspects of REM sleep are so typical of wakefulness, there are some distinct differences. For example, neurons using the neurotransmitter noradrenaline, and very active during wakefulness, are quite inactive during REM sleep. However, this difference has to be weighed against the other, impressive similarities between wakefulness and REM sleep.

I likened REM sleep to a computer in 'screen-saver' mode, with the computer occupying itself, still running but not switched off. A quick touch of the keyboard instantly brings it back to life. Extending this computer analogy to deep sleep, here the computer is turned off, needing to be 'booted up'—which takes a little time before it becomes fully functional and 'awake'.

If REM sleep is so much like wakefulness, maybe it can, at least in part, be replaced by wakefulness, which seems to happen during our first year of life, when there is a rapid decline in this type of sleep—seemingly replaced by wakefulness. However, substitution of REM sleep by wakefulness is not a simple matter. If we are woken up whenever REM sleep appears, and kept awake for just a few minutes, we are noticeably sleepier in the day, having clearly lost out on sleep. Such wakefulness is no substitute for REM sleep. On the other hand, if we keep awake for longer, during what would have been a full bout of REM sleep—say, for about 15 minutes or so—there seems to be less of an effect on daytime sleepiness, even after a couple of nights of this regimen.[1] Furthermore, there is only a small increase in REM sleep on the recovery night—much less than the REM sleep that was lost. These latter clues suggest that at least some of REM sleep and wakefulness might be interchangeable.[2]

Let us follow this line of thinking a bit further. The atonia or paralysis experienced during REM sleep indicates that we may need to move, but the actual movement has to be blocked, for safety and other reasons. Nevertheless, it seems that some aspect of movement is important to REM sleep. What would happen if, during the deprivation of REM sleep, we did not just lie in bed, but got up and walked about energetically to simulate the intended movement within REM sleep? Unfortunately, this simple study has yet to be done in humans, although there are findings[2] with laboratory rats, where REM sleep is deprived by gentle methods, in particular through playful handling. Subsequently (within limits), there is no rebound increase in REM sleep when the animal is eventually allowed recovery sleep. Similarly, when cats are woken from REM sleep, and gently handled for around six minutes (the average length of a period of REM sleep in a cat), there is neither any change to waking behaviour nor any subsequent rebound in REM sleep, suggesting that the wakefulness had somehow substituted for the missing REM sleep. However, I am cautious about all this, because such findings with animals need much more investigation.

So, why would the brain apparently want us to move about during

REM sleep, only to suppress the movement with paralysis? Why not just have nil intended movement, as happens with the rest of sleep, when we simply lie down and sleep without the paralysis? Maybe this apparent need for movement in REM sleep is a carry-over from the time before birth, when movement helped the baby to develop the connections between its brain and limb muscles, but with actual movement constrained by the confines of the uterus. Besides, lots of real movement would cause the mother much discomfort. So, perhaps the huge amount of REM sleep in the pre-term baby substitutes for this movement by allowing it to 'go through the motions' so to speak.

Could the apparently blocked emotions during our REM sleep have a similar role for the baby—in allowing it to 'blow off steam' within the frustrating confines of the uterus? Maybe this continues in the adult, with REM sleep acting as some sort of emotional safety valve? However, before coming to a more Freudian interpretation of REM sleep, we must ask why are those antidepressant medicines that knock out REM sleep so successful? Surely they would just increase emotional frustration—which they do not. And what about that happy, well-balanced, friendly dolphin with no REM sleep at all?

Yet, the similarities between REM sleep and wakefulness are remarkable and, apart from our being unconscious during REM sleep, I believe that it can be likened to a form of wakefulness rather than a true sleep, typified by non-REM sleep. Through being so evident and intense towards the end of sleep, just before normal waking, REM sleep seems, at least, to be preparing us for wakefulness. To these ends we might consider REM sleep not as 'real sleep' but as wakefulness being switched off rather than 'true sleep' being switched on, as happens with non-REM sleep—that is, REM sleep is a screen-saving 'non-wakefulness'.

Thus, whatever functions REM sleep may have, we need to look back to our early life within the uterus, as we have so much of it then and there, where the developing brain needs waking-like sensory bombardment, and to make up for its absence we have REM sleep. Moreover, this developing infant probably needs to 'exercise its muscles' or at least to try to, but is physically restricted from doing so—and here is where REM sleep steps in again. As the emotional centres of this brain are also developing, maybe REM sleep provides an 'emotional sponge'. For us adults, retaining lesser amounts of REM sleep, maybe it fulfils similar functions, whereby the truly sleeping brain periodically becomes 'bored' and in need of the activities of REM sleep, with dreaming being a further attempt to provide this, by turning all that 'pseudo-sensory bombardment' into the 'cinema of the mind'.

More on memory

Rapid eye movement sleep was once thought to play a vital role in memory by somehow sorting out the days events and loading the important material into more permanent memories, throwing out the rubbish as dreams—as the mind's junkyard. However, this idea cannot explain the lack of any memory impairment following the suppression of REM sleep by those antidepressant drugs. Undaunted, others have undertaken many experiments to see whether intense daytime learning affects REM sleep. The most interesting findings are that areas of the brain stimulated by learning when we are awake also become active in REM sleep. This is not to say that REM sleep is intimately involved in the laying down of memories, because there is an alternative explanation, from my perspective, that REM sleep is like wakefulness. It is simply that memories utilised in wakefulness are revived in similar ways during REM sleep—why not if it is akin to wakefulness? Maybe this just contributes to the manufacture of dreams, given that we tend to dream about what happened the previous day, and in doing so revive these memories, albeit in a jumbled way. Findings that parts of the brain active during waking learning are active again in REM sleep do not point to some unique, essential memory processing during REM sleep. It is rather like the rapid eye movements of REM sleep, which are just like those of wakefulness, although REM sleep does not provide the eyes with any unique benefit, because the loss of REM sleep, together with its eye movements, has no ill-effect on the ability to see.

Recent sophisticated ('gene expression') studies on rats have looked at whether long periods (for example, ten days) of REM sleep deprivation cause brain impairment, but nothing of note has been found. Earlier claims that, for the rat, REM sleep somehow offers unique benefits to its learning were largely based on stressful REM sleep deprivation experiments, where the animal sits on a raised platform, surrounded by water, is liable to fall in, and is very exposed because it cannot run off and hide.[2] The stress imposed on these animals is probably more than that for any accompanying 'stress control' animal, which is able to snatch some sleep and less likely to fall into the water. Stress, rather than the loss of REM sleep itself, causes rats to change their behaviour, because they become more aggressive and fearful, which must also interfere with their ability to learn.

Having said this, I mentioned in Chapter 2 that 'procedural memory', linked to the learning of new skills and habits (for example, riding a bike, playing a musical instrument, playing a new game of cards) that we are not consciously aware of, which somehow improve with practice, may obtain some benefit from REM sleep. These are largely skills involving movement and maybe the paralysed movement during REM sleep has a part to play here? On the other hand, it may just be another example of REM sleep being like wakefulness and simply 'copying' waking activities in some way. Whatever the role of REM sleep in procedural memory, it is probably minor at best, and for those interested in this topic I refer you to the insightful critique of REM sleep and memory,[3] written by the astute Dr Jerry Siegel, from the University of California at Los Angeles. I defer to his conclusion[3] that the 'existing literature does not indicate a major role for REM sleep in memory consolidation' (p 1063).

Fear

I suspect, however, that REM sleep helps some animals, especially rats and mice, to cope with stress or, more to the point, fear. This is unlikely to be so much the case with humans because we have other, more sophisticated ways of dealing with it. There are many rat studies showing that stressing situations apart from the 'platform methods' just mentioned, such as (painlessly) immobilising the animal in a humane trap, placing it in the open where it cannot run off and hide, or exposing it to threats from other animals, usually lead to particularly large increases in REM sleep. Stress is an acceptable term to use here, but fear is not, because without being able to communicate with the animal we do not really know what it feels. But let us be bold and call it fear, nevertheless.

If these same animals are also deprived of sleep (including REM sleep, of course), then they are dealt a double blow, because they are deprived of a way by which they cope with the stress—in not having REM sleep. Together, these two factors (that is, stress plus no REM sleep) may explain why these animals have particular learning difficulties, as learning some pointless task is, to say the least, low on their priorities. 'Stress control' animals in these studies may well be similarly stressed, but as they are allowed REM sleep the situation is more tolerable. The huge increase ('rebound') of REM sleep appearing when the sleep-deprived animals are allowed recovery sleep is, I believe, a stress-cum-fear coping response. If they are deprived of REM sleep in a gentler, more tender way, there is little learning deficit or much by way of an REM sleep rebound afterwards.[2]

By the way, we do not have increased REM sleep when stressed. If anything, there is more fitful sleep with less REM sleep. The latter does not show much rebound when the stress is over—seemingly what REM sleep was lost has gone for good.

A disorder of sleep or of wakefulness?

An abnormal and sudden onset of what often (but not always) appears to be REM sleep during wakefulness is seen in the neurological disorder, narcolepsy, found in at least some form in about one in 600 people. Although it can have a hereditary basis, this is not always the case, because only one of a pair of identical twins might suffer. It usually appears after adolescence, and unusually after the mid-30s. The most obvious symptoms are excessive sleepiness (especially during monotony and boredom), and 'sleep attacks' with little or no forewarning. Often, when sufferers take a voluntary nap or go to sleep at night, they are more likely than usual to enter REM sleep rapidly, and can have what is known as a 'sleep-onset REM period'— SOREMP for short—which can be of diagnostic help, but not always.

Most sufferers with narcolepsy also have 'cataplexy' when fully awake, which is a sudden weakness over all or part of the body (usually the legs), brought on by sudden emotional excitement, such as anger, laughter, surprise, or even watching an exciting sporting event. Weakness can last from seconds up to a minute, and may involve a total or partial collapse (of just the legs), which can be quite wrongly mistaken for a faint or fit, except that they remain conscious, with open eyes that are still able to move about at will. Inasmuch as many of us go 'weak at the knees' when we laugh, maybe cataplexy is just a more extreme form of this reaction. Some have argued that cataplexy might have had survival value in ancient times, in causing the individual to 'play possum' and pretend to be dead. As many predators want to kill their own prey rather than eat already dead meat, they pass by. However, this is hardly a very comforting thought for present-day sufferers.

Sometimes this cataplexy quickly develops into a narcoleptic 'sleep attack', typically with REM sleep rapidly appearing, but not always, because this sleep may consist only of non-REM sleep. There may also be an accompanying vivid dream-like imagery. These sleep attacks last for about ten minutes, when the sufferer will wake up spontaneously, albeit somewhat confused.

Other symptoms of narcolepsy, usually found after lights out at night when going to sleep, include vivid visual hallucinations (which seem to be dream intrusions into wakefulness), and body paralysis—similar to that of REM sleep itself. This is a more serious case of the 'sleep paralysis' mentioned earlier. In these patients, the paralysis and hallucinations can reappear on awakening the next morning. Episodes, such as those before sleep, last for around five minutes and can be quite frightening. Extreme fright can play tricks on the mind. For example, during the First World War, when soldiers were waiting for the 'whistle to blow', ordering them 'over the top' of the trenches to confront enemy machine guns and maybe get killed, there were many reports of 'out-of-body experiences'. They would somehow see themselves, detached from their bodies and from some distance away. I mention this because it is not 'spooky', but maybe a way in which the mind can handle fear. This sensation is also sometimes experienced by patients with narcolepsy during episodes of hallucinatory sleep paralysis, and is not a sign of their going mad.

Narcoleptic sleep attacks in the day worsen sleep quality at night, which is mostly why patients also suffer from fitful night-time sleep. Some also find that they may become very forgetful, but this apparent memory problem is probably not caused by the disorder itself, or by disruptions to REM sleep.

Treatment of narcolepsy–cataplexy is 'symptomatic'—that is, some of the symptoms can be controlled to varying extents by drugs—but neither the narcolepsy nor the cataplexy can be cured. The daytime sleepiness can be treated by stimulants or stimulant-like medicines to suppress the sleepiness, and the cataplexy can be helped by drugs that suppress REM sleep—even the (non-sedating) antidepressants that I mentioned earlier. Most patients find that by taking pre-emptive short naps in the day, they can reduce or fend off unwanted sleep attacks. One stimulant-like medicine (modafinil, with the proprietary name Provigil®) is remarkable in that it still allows people to nap and, combined with additional treatment for cataplexy, patients can be helped considerably. Nevertheless, narcolepsy–cataplexy is a debilitating illness, and perhaps the only good news at the moment is that it is not life shortening, provided that serious accidents do not happen because of the sleep attacks. Many undiagnosed patients become quite depressed by the illness, and the doctor who misses the correct diagnosis may think that depression is the actual cause and prescribe antidepressants. The improvement of the cataplexy, which follows, may simply reinforce the doctor's wrong diagnosis.

There are more promising treatments on the horizon that may well centre on the discovery of the brain substance, orexin–hypocretin. Recently, it was noticed, in studies of appetite in rodents, that animals with very low levels of this substance also had sleep attacks. On further investigation, it turned out to be a form of narcolepsy. Injections of orexin–hypocretin increased the animals' alertness and suppressed the propensity to sleep. Moreover, it is now known that most humans with narcolepsy have an orexin–hypocretin deficiency, although not all of them, which means that this is not the root cause of narcolepsy–cataplexy but is somehow tied in to it. As orexin–hypocretin also affects appetite, eating behaviour, and metabolism, it suggests that REM sleep may be linked in with these other functions, in tantalising ways that are not yet understood.

By the way, patients with narcolepsy can experience food cravings, although the actual link with narcolepsy may be more complicated than at first might seem.

In a nutshell

This account of REM sleep is a patchwork of selected views of other researchers stitched into my own collage, which I hope presents a more complete, albeit rather controversial picture. In particular my approach to REM sleep has been stimulated by the work of Professor Michel Jouvet, the doyen of sleep research, to whom we owe so much, who described REM (paradoxical) sleep as 'archisleep'—the earliest form of sleep to evolve, both in terms of evolution and foetal life (although its characteristics do change during brain development).

Although I do not wish to be repetitive, I would like to summarise the points: during REM sleep there is awareness of the environment, to the extent that the brain can decide whether or not to wake up. We can rouse rapidly from this sleep, more so than from most of non-REM sleep. During REM sleep the brain is bombarded by numerous artificial sensations coming from within, helping to keep it preoccupied and distracting us from waking. These would normally cause us to move around and experience emotions, and so both must be blocked, otherwise we would keep waking up—hence the paralysis, and why the accompanying emotional feelings are absent, leaving us in a detached frame of mind, unless things become really bad as in a nightmare. Although dreaming helps the brain make some sense of this bombardment, dreams keep jumping from one unexpected and unrelated event to another, probably because the part of the brain, the frontal cortex, that stops us from being continually side tracked like this is switched off or is resting in some way during REM sleep. It is probably why, in our dreams, we cannot focus on a more predictable and consistent theme. On the other hand, all this unexpectedness makes them all the more fascinating and distracts us from pointlessly waking up.

Rapid eye movement sleep is prevalent in early intrauterine development, where the stimulation that it provides probably helps with brain development in the absence of real sensory stimulation.

Whether or not babies dream to any extent is something that we will probably never know. In the adult, REM sleep also helps keep the brain 'tweaked up' and prepared for wakefulness. Moreover, much of REM sleep may act as a substitute for wakefulness not only in the baby, but also in the adult. This may account for why it has features similar to wakefulness and less like those of non-REM sleep, with the latter having more of the qualities of a real recovery state for the brain. This is why I liken REM sleep to wakefulness being switched off, rather than sleep being switched on. It is not so much a form of sleep, but a state of 'non-wakefulness', quickly and easily reversible to wakefulness, which, again, is uncharacteristic of non-REM sleep.

And finally . . .

Sleep and wakefulness are not 'opposites', with one just being the absence of the other. They are complementary states working in harmony, as well as with other bodily needs such as feeding. Sleep and wakefulness tend to be controlled by separate parts of the brain, and I think that it is helpful to see each of them as being on or off, making four combinations in all. Whereas REM sleep is where I propose that both sleep and wakefulness are switched 'off' (as 'non-wakefulness'), non-REM sleep is 'true' sleep, with wakefulness 'off' and sleep 'on'. Alert wakefulness is, of course, wake 'on' and sleep 'off'. What about the final combination, both sleep and wakefulness being on together? I see this as drowsiness. Many mammals, especially farm animals, spend much of the day 'suspended' in this state, which has perplexed many sleep researchers as to what it is. Is it sleep or is it wakefulness? Well, it is probably both! As to whether or how the brain or even the body might benefit from drowsiness still remains a mystery, but this state still allows the animal to remain somewhat vigilant to danger, and maybe its cortex can obtain some rest—who knows? Let me summarise these four combinations as in Table 2.

Lastly, again, I have to say how ironic it is that not only is most of sleep non-REM sleep, identified by something that it is not, but that, by implication, REM sleep is the centre of the sleep universe, so to

Table 2 Four combinations of sleep and wakefulness

	Wakefulness system	Sleep system
Alert	+	−
Drowsy	+	+
Non-REM sleep	−	+
REM sleep	−	−

speak—which it is not. In fact, for us, the real crux of sleep probably lies in those really slow brain waves of deep non-REM sleep.

Cinema of the mind

Imagery

Whereas the mental activity of rapid eye movement (REM) sleep is intense, visual, and florid, more tranquil thoughts and imagery do occur during the rest of sleep, which sleep researchers refer to as 'thinking' or 'mentation'. Sometimes, however, what appears to be real dreaming can be found in non-REM sleep. Other interesting visual states exist in and around sleep for some people, who have the ability to conjure up visual scenes during drowsiness and light sleep. This reverie is called 'hypnagogic' imagery when it occurs around sleep onset and 'hypnopompic' imagery during morning awakening. Although having different names, both seem to be the same phenomenon, and are derived from the Greek *hypnos* (sleep), *agogos* (leads), and *apophysis* (outgrowth). Some conscious control can be exerted here, and a few people can maintain these pleasant states for many minutes. Children seem particularly good at it, and this may be one reason why bedtime stories can be so enrapturing for them—they can easily visualise what is going on in the fairy tales. Less pleasant states, such as sleepwalking and the alarming 'sleep terror', are aberrant features of deep non-REM sleep, whereas the more benign sleep talking is usually associated with light sleep. I explain more about these conditions in Chapter 22 when I come to children's sleep, because it is in children rather than adults in whom these strange states are more likely to occur.

Back to dreaming—as in REM sleep. Some people claim to be aware that they are dreaming and consciously manipulate their dreams. Called 'lucid dreaming', it still remains a puzzle, but at least some of it is mistaken for the imagery just mentioned. Although many of us do become more aware of dreaming towards the conclusion of a dream, just before waking, it is another matter whether it can be manipulated to our own ends. Whereas some dream researchers believe that most of us can train ourselves to become lucid dreamers, or control our dreams better, many others doubt it.

The ability to recall dreams on awakening in the morning is very limited because the memory of dreams soon evaporates. Recall is best if one wakes or is awoken directly from a dream, because waking up five minutes into light sleep, after a dream, produces only fragmented accounts, and after ten minutes there is little or no recall. The reason why some people are good at remembering their dreams is usually because they wake up periodically during the night, often from their dreams—maybe because they are poor or fitful sleepers. Recalling the dream during this brief wakefulness makes it more easily recounted later.

Absence of any knowledge of dreaming may simply be a sign of good and undisturbed sleep. Studies of people who claim never to dream find that, when they have their EEGs recorded, and are awoken after ten minutes or so of REM sleep, to their amazement, they usually admit to having been dreaming. On the other hand, it seems that, for all of us, about one in five awakenings from REM sleep produces no dream reports—which means either no dreaming or that the dream was rapidly forgotten.

Some 2,000 years ago Aristotle, in his treatise *Parva Naturalia*,[1] gave an insightful account of how dreams are formed, after dismissing the current view of the time that they were 'sent by the gods'. Dreams, he surmised, were mostly based on residual images left in the mind from various events previously seen or thought about. These presented themselves: 'with even greater impression . . . like little eddies which are being formed in rivers . . . often remaining like what they were when they first started, but often, too, broken into other forms by collisions. . . . If one violently disturbs these residuary movements they become confused . . . this may occur particularly in people who are atrabilious, or feverish, or intoxicated'.

It is clear that not only do dreams include some of the previous day's visual happenings, but also sounds and other harmless noises can be incorporated. Even gentle spraying of water onto the skin can produce dreams involving water. In contrast, when this spray is given in non-REM sleep, there are no reports of 'thinking about water'. Alarm clocks going off can also become incorporated into ongoing dreams, usually as a doorbell or phone.

Fascinating facts

Nine out of ten dreams seem to involve the dreamers themselves in bizarre everyday life events. Men are more likely to dream about other men than women, whereas for women it is equally about both sexes. Interestingly, most of the characters in our dreams are unrecognisable and they are seldom famous people. For both men and women, around half the social interactions in dreams seem to be aggressive, usually directed towards the dreamer. However, our responses in these dreams usually involve apprehension and confusion rather than panic or fright. I mentioned in Chapter 15 that there are rarely any real emotions behind these sensations, because they seem to be switched off. Any aggression in a dream is rarely violent, but usually verbal or by gestures, and hardly ever sexual. Whereas about a third of dreams convey misfortune, few are of good fortune. About half the settings for dreams are unknown, about a quarter are known locations, and for the remainder the setting is hazy. Eating spicy or indigestible foods at night does not make us dream more, but simply disturbs sleep and makes it more likely that we wake up out of a dream.

We are not alone as dreamers—remember those cats without the normal paralysis of REM sleep described earlier, which were clearly enacting their dreams? Many dog owners watching Fido sleeping in front of the fire will often see periodic twitching and yelping—a close-up look at the eyes will show them periodically darting about under the eyelids. However, we must not assume that their dreams are mostly visual images, because dogs rely heavily on thier sense of smell. Chimpanzees, like us, rely heavily on vision, and Washoe, the famous chimpanzee who was taught sign language and able to communicate with her keepers, often combined the symbols for 'sleep' and 'pictures'. Whereas Aristotle believed that dreaming was confined to 'all four legged animals', Charles Darwin was quite adamant that birds have vivid dreams, because he noted that when sleeping on their perches they periodically 'chirruped'—but maybe they were just getting more comfortable!

We are usually the centrepiece of our dreams, albeit somehow detached and watching from a different perspective than 'through our own eyes', but it is not like an 'out of body experience'. This could be a reason behind the belief of some more primitive cultures that one's soul leaves the body during dreaming and goes on its travels. In this instance, waking someone up suddenly had to be avoided at all costs because it could prevent the soul returning in time. For about 20 years, from the mid-1930s, Dr Kilton Stewart periodically lived with a primitive tribe of people called the Senoi, who inhabited the deep Malayan jungle. He sent back various reports claiming that these people devoted much time each day to discussing and sharing their dreams, and where they had visited in their dreams. Dreams guided their waking behaviour. So, for example, if they had upset someone in their dream they would make it up to them the next day. Moreover, if they had been upset by someone else in this dream, they would inform that person and expect to be treated particularly well by them![2]

Stewart claimed that, as a result of their dream experiences, these people had no mental illness and they were very happy, peaceful, and content. The publicity given by the media to this utopian society soon caught on in the USA, especially in the more enlightened 1960s, and various therapies based on this approach to dreaming emerged. Articles even appeared in medical and scientific journals about the benefits of the therapy. Alas, the bubble burst some 20 years later in an exposé by Dr William Domhoff, in his book *The Mystique of Dreams*.[3] The rather over-zealous Stewart seemed to have added his own embellishments to his writings, because the Senoi spent no more time discussing their dreams than anyone else. There was mental illness in the tribe and they were no more peaceful and happy than any other native peoples. It makes a good story though and, I suspect, provides us with another lesson on the pitfalls of dream research.

Events in dreams seem to run their full course, in the same time it would take to visualise the experiences in wakefulness. There is little support for the idea that dreams are all over in a 'flash' or are substantially compressed in time. This latter notion was challenged as early as 1897 by a Dr J. Claviere who took as one example the famous dream of a fellow Frenchman, Maury, who was awoken by a board falling on his neck. Maury recounted a long story of events in his dream that ended in him being guillotined—that is, when the board fell. Therefore, Maury argued, the whole dream must have been constructed the instant the board fell, but Claviere doubted the accuracy of the account.

People woken up between about 5 and 15 minutes into a period of REM sleep (as measured by the EEG), and asked to say for how long they thought that they had been dreaming, have a pretty good idea of the duration. On the other hand, if they are woken at the end of a more lengthy period of REM sleep, their accounts seem no longer than for about 15 minutes—the early part is apparently forgotten. Thus, the extent of dream recall is limited to about this length of time, which must make attempts at dream interpretation difficult for dreams in excess of 15 minutes. It is like trying to understand the plot of a good novel without knowing the beginning, only the end.

Children under five seldom report dreaming even when woken out of REM sleep, and then only to report rather dull goings on. From five to nine years of age, dreams seem to become more as we know them, but usually do not involve the dreamer—more likely animals! Few children's dreams seem to involve school or TV characters, but are more likely to include enjoyable play activities. Of course, children are less adept at using words, which probably constrains what they really experience in the dream. The more the child is prompted over what the dream is about, the more forthcoming he or she may be, but it is likely that at least some of this prompting simply puts more ideas into the mind and the child confabulates.

Difficulties

Dreams are usually visual, which is not surprising when one considers that vision is by far our dominant sense. We usually dream in colour, and those who claim to dream only in black and white usually have a hazy recollection of their dream because too much time has elapsed between the dream and its recollection—hence the colours have faded in the 'mind's eye'. For people born blind or who lose their sight before about the age of five, dreaming is mostly in the form of sounds and voices, and to a lesser extent touch, taste, and smell. Whereas there are few rapid eye movements during REM sleep for those who are blind from birth, such eye movements are quite apparent with a later onset of blindness. Many blind people dream a lot about their guide dogs.

The problem with studying the dreams of other people is that we have no idea of the extent to which these are an accurate reflection of what was dreamt, or unwittingly embellished or perhaps knowingly censored by the dreamer. Ask several alert people to watch a short film and then to recount what they saw. Although some of the exciting parts will be remembered more accurately, even these recollections will vary—and, as for the more incidental scenes, well that is anyone's guess. Dreams, similar to these films, are visual, whereas the recounting of both is verbal or written, and it is difficult for some people verbally to recount or write down complex scenes, especially if these are fading rapidly from memory.

Many exponents of dream analysis give up at this point and simply concentrate on their own personal dreams. This might seem a good idea because the 'middle man' is eliminated, so to speak. On the other hand, the dreaming 'self' might decide that it does not want the dream interpreted and distort the dream even more, so that the waking 'self' is put off the scent or left completely baffled by these mind games! As each of us has difficulty in recalling any dream, because the image soon evaporates, and as there are so many more dreams that we have forgotten, any potentially revealing information from a dream is seldom evident. Of course, it might be argued that the dreams that we remember are only the important ones!

More scientifically oriented dream researchers bring their sleepers into the laboratory, to monitor their EEGs and wake them up from REM sleep. Sounds good, but as these sleepers are also usually forewarned about this being a study of dreaming, it is not surprising that about a quarter of these dreams centre on the laboratory itself. At least the recollection of these dreams is more systematically recorded than the spontaneous dream recollections that one has at home, which are probably biased towards those dreams having greater impact—one easily forgets a dull dream. Another technique—of phoning up a volunteer at home, randomly, in the middle of the night and asking them immediately what was going on in their sleeping mind—sounds a good idea, but the odds are that they would not be woken out of REM sleep or, if one was lucky and hit REM sleep, the dream might have only just begun.

Such problems illustrate why I do not study dreams, but sit on the sideline and watch the dream researchers often arguing among themselves. Dreams should be treated as the cinema of the mind, fictitious and purely for entertainment. Besides, most are only poor quality 'B movies'—best forgotten, anyway!

Interpretation

What is fairly clear is that we dream as we think—dreams are a surreal pastiche of what we have recently encountered and thought about during wakefulness. Why people want to place some meaning into dreams or 'interpret' them is beyond the comprehension of many of us, and probably beyond the understanding of those many people who write about the meaning of dreams. There is usually greater fantasy emanating from the mind of the dream interpreter than from the dream to be interpreted. Nevertheless, this has been a focus of countless writings since writing began. The Greeks and Romans placed much significance in dreams, as shown in the five volumes of *Oneirocritica*, written by Artemidorus in around AD 120. Over 3,000 dream accounts were given, with the translation of numerous dream symbols (for example, the right hand = father, son or friend; left hand = mother, wife or mistress; foot = slave; a dolphin in water = good omen; one out of water = bad omen). Artemidorus wisely insisted that dreams be interpreted in relation to each dreamer, his or her customs, and where he or she lives. This is why dream interpretation was so difficult, and apparently could be left to only a few informed individuals. Even Sigmund Freud was impressed by these writings, and often referred to Artemidorus.

Viewing dreams as portents of the future has been another popular approach for dream 'interpreters'. The ancient Egyptians developed dream interpretation into both an art and a religion. Priests would conduct their interpretations as part of sleep therapy carried out in 'sleep temples'. There is an ancient papyrus, the *Dream Book*, from the era of Ramses the Second (1275 BCE), in the British Museum, and it provides numerous dream examples and interpretations. People with troubled minds would spend the night in these special temples where priests would try to influence sleep with suggestions in the hope of provoking special dreams sent by the gods. In fact, Imhotep, the architect of the first step pyramid and a famous physician of the time, advocated this practice. After his death he was worshipped as a god, in sleep temples built in his honour. In ancient Greece this same practice was adopted for many years until the fourth century BP, with the god of healing, Asclepios, acquiring the role of Imhotep. Some hundreds of years later, the sceptical Aristotle had more insightful comments to make in his *Parva Naturalia*, where he wrote, 'most prophetic dreams are . . . mere coincidences'.[1] But he pointed out that dreams can subconsciously change behaviour and bring about a foreseen event: 'for as when we are engaged on any course of action, or have performed certain actions . . . the dream movement has had a way paved for it, which in turn should prove a starting point for action to be performed'.[1] He also noted that:

> The most skilful interpreter of dreams is he who has the faculty of observing resemblances. Anyone may interpret dreams which are vivid and plain. But . . . dreams are analogous to forms reflected in water . . . if the motion in the water is great, the reflection has no resemblance to the original. Skilful is he who could rapidly discern . . . the rapid and distorted fragments . . . for internal movements efface the clearness of dreams.

It is possible that in certain situations dreams can be of help in understanding the pressures that confront patients with severe mental problems, and to some extent Freud may have been correct in saying that dreams are the 'royal road to the unconscious'. But to endorse Artemidorus's point, it is crucial to know the patient before any 'interpretation' can begin, and there is no evidence to support the notion of universal symbols in dream imagery, common to humankind. 'Dream dictionaries' and schemes for 'dream analyses by mail', where there is no rapport between the dreamer and interpreter, must be treated with the greatest of suspicion.

Freud's views on the interpretation of dreams are highly contentious, of course, particularly because of their highly sexual bias. Interestingly, and much to his disappointment, his now famous book
Interpretation of Dreams was very dull and turgid in its original version,
only selling 351 copies in its first six years. So he wrote a more popular
account, and the rest is history. It is the latter, more sensational version that caused several of his followers to go off to create their own
schemes for dream interpretation. Subsequently, a somewhat dis-
heartened Freud wrote in his *New Introductory Lectures on
Psychoanalysis*:

> . . . but if you ask how much of dream interpretation has been accepted by
> outsiders, by the many psychiatrists and psychotherapists who warm their
> pot of soup at our fire (incidentally without being very grateful for our
> hospitality), by what are described as educated people, who are in the habit
> of assimilating the more striking findings of science, by the literary men
> and by the public at large—the reply gives little cause for satisfaction. (p 8)[4]

Dream interpretation is one matter and the role of dreams another.
Freud could well be right in saying that dreams were 'wish fulfil-
ments', to provide a substitute way for discharging repressed emotions
or unconscious wishes. These feelings are probably not as sexually
oriented as Freud suggested, but are more diverse, as most modern
psychoanalysts believe. Nevertheless, Freud had a remarkable insight
into dreaming, in particular that at least two types of mental activity
seem to be going on, which he describes as the 'manifest' and the
'latent' contents of the dream. The latter is an expression of basic
biological drives (which for Freud were mainly sexual), which may be
too emotive for the sleeper to handle, and this is where a form of
censor within the mind comes in, to moderate the offending parts
and to produce the 'manifest' dream. Freud explained several mechanisms by which the manifest dream was produced, such as 'conden-
sation'—the clustering of several meanings into an image—and 'dis-
placement'—the shifting of emotionally painful experiences onto a
more benign image.

One has to remember that in Freud's time there was a socially
repressive society where convention demanded that true feelings
be hidden. Thus, dreams were probably the only method by which

feelings could be expressed, albeit in a distorted way. Today, in a liberated society we can be more open with our emotions, and maybe our dreams are less tortuous and more pleasant and entertaining. Thus, contemporary psychotherapists inclined towards dream interpretation might better spend their time assessing the depths of the waking mind rather than delving into dreams.

What impressed Freud, and many others (myself included), is how remarkably elaborate dreams are for most people. He also noted 'we have found evidence in the dream, thoughts of a highly complex intellectual function, operating with almost the whole resources of the mental apparatus'.[4] Dreaming becomes even more awesome when one considers how it is almost impossible during wakefulness for most of us to produce such colourful and complex scenarios from within our imagination, lasting for half an hour or so.

Freud also saw the dream as the 'guardian of sleep', and in this respect so did his contemporary, Dr Carl Jung, who, like Freud, also thought dreams had a compensatory function. Through their content and release of emotions, Jung proposed that, 'dreams contribute to the self-regulation of the psyche'.[5] For Jung, however, dreams were the expression of the 'collective unconscious . . . that lies at a deeper level and is further removed from consciousness than the personal unconscious . . . in the dream the psyche speaks in images and gives expression to instincts which derive from the most primitive levels of nature'.[5]

If typical dreaming is largely confined to REM sleep, what happens to dreaming when REM sleep is removed for long periods of time, with antidepressant treatment, for example? Does the REM-less dolphin dream? No one really knows—maybe dreaming shifts into non-REM sleep, or we experience more dream-like fantasising during wakefulness? More radical views, and perhaps not what one might expect from Nathaniel Kleitman, the co-discoverer of REM sleep (as we know it today), are not fondly remembered by many dream researchers, because he cynically dismissed dreaming by likening it to vomiting.

To those who insist that because dreams occur they must serve a particular purpose, it may be pointed out that not all processes have a teleological explanation. Vomiting, for instance, when it is elicited by some irritating matter in the stomach, serves a good purpose in evacuating the stomach and removing the irritant. The same vomiting act, when resulting from motion sickness, serves no physiological purpose. . . . As such, dreaming sleep need not have any special function and may be quite meaningless. (p 107)[6]

One can only hope that Kleitman derived some pleasure from his dreams, rather than having nightmares about vomit. Kleitman might have been prosaic in dismissing the significance of dreams, but he was not poetic about it, as was Geoffrey Chaucer, whose thoughts might be equally astute but more palatable, as in this little ditty from the *Priest's Tale*:

> For dreams are but vanities and japes
> Men dream every day of owls and apes.
> And with many a nonsense of all of this.
> They dream of what has never been and never is.[7]

Depressing dreams

On a more serious note, I would like to return briefly to the topic of depression, and the fact that many of the most effective drugs available to treat depression also suppress REM sleep. In doing so, they probably knock out much of the more vivid forms of dreaming. This suppression of REM sleep is immediate and happens on the first night after taking the tablets, unlike the improvement to the depression itself, which can take several weeks. Whether these medicines partly work through the suppression of REM sleep and dreaming remains a matter for debate, especially as they have other beneficial effects unrelated to REM sleep. However, I suspect that there is a connection. For example, if we do indeed 'dream as we think', then, given that depressed people tend to have miserable waking thoughts, the same will happen to their dreams. Although they have little recollection of these or any other dreams in the morning, these sad dreams may leave a residual sadness on awakening, which carries on into the day. Coincidentally or otherwise, many sufferers of depression do feel worse in the mornings and, to come to my point, removal of these sad dreams may allow one at least to begin the day in a somewhat better frame of mind and, if continued day after day, the effect may become more sustained.

The future

The notion that dreams are omens to the future, if only one could get the interpretation right, still persists to the present day. The difficulty is that, as we have many dreams each night, who knows which might be portentous, because they all cannot be so. What is more, owing to the randomness of dreams one is bound to strike lucky now and again through pure chance. This is illustrated by the desperate attempts to find the 20-month-old son of Charles Lindberg (the famous trans-Atlantic aviator), who was kidnapped in March 1932, but, tragically, discovered buried a few miles away two months later, killed soon after the kidnapping. The kidnapper, eventually identified as Bruno Hauptmann, had seemingly sent nine ransom notes, and the media were in a frenzy. Advertisements were put in newspapers asking for help from anyone claiming to have prophetic dreams as to the where-abouts of the baby. Well over 1,000 dream reports were received. A subsequent analysis of these showed only seven to have anything near to the truth and none was spot on. By the way, although Haupt-mann was arrested, convicted, and executed for the crime, many doubted his guilt.

Arguably the biggest study into dream premonitions was under-taken some 40 years later by the science editor of the London news-paper, the *Evening Standard*. He invited readers to send in accounts of their more spectacular dreams, as soon as they happened. Attempts were then made to match these up with subsequent news stories. This continued for 15 years, with thousands of dream accounts amassed. Although some did seem to ring true, this was no greater than would have been the case by chance.

On a final and more positive note, dreams can be delightful and inspirational. Leonardo da Vinci attributed many of his inventions to dreams and wrote, 'why does the eye see a thing more clearly in dreams than the imagination when awake?'.[8] Elias Howe, the inventor of the sewing machine, is said to have dreamt the inspir-ation of a needle with its thread hole near to its tip. James Watt invented the steam engine, but he also invented what is still the process for making lead shot, which came to him in a recurrent dream. In it he was walking along in heavy rain, coming down as hard pellets. He experimented for real, by pouring molten lead from a church tower into a water-filled moat below—it worked! Freidrich Kékulé, the discoverer of organic chemistry and the benzene ring, attributed his inspiration to a dream of a snake swallowing its tail. Robert Louis Stevenson frequently had vivid dreams, and his most famous story 'The Strange Case of Dr Jekyll and Mr Hyde' came from a dream, as did some of the most important features of the tale, such as the use of the evil potion. Although Samuel Taylor Coleridge's 'Kubla Khan' was supposed to be inspired by his dreams, his smoking of opium was the more likely cause! Sadly, not all dreams are so benign and useful, especially when coming from national leaders, such as Bismarck, whose plan for nineteenth-century Europe was attributed to his having dreamt about it. This was one dream that he should have forgotten.

17 The long, the short, and the less

Normal sleepers

With good sleepers of any age there will be some who naturally sleep longer or shorter than the average, and I am excluding those who have insomnia. For adults aged between 20 and 70 years, the average sleep is between 7 and 8 hours a night, and this is what we[1] found in our study of 400 people (see Chapter 12). In fact, the average sleep length was about 7 hours 10 minutes for men and 7 hours 30 minutes for women. Women reporting sleeping around 20 minutes longer than men is a common finding worldwide. Figure 15 shows the distribution of this sleep for all our participants, who reported their nightly sleep lengths for a total of 5,718 nights out of the possible 6,000. Around this 7–8 hours average is the typical bell-shaped 'normal distribution', with decreasing numbers sleeping longer and shorter than

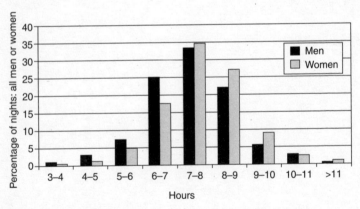

Figure 15 Hours slept at night.

this average. Whereas about 34 per cent of the nights were between 7 and 8 hours, almost 80 per cent were between 6 and 9 hours, leaving 20 per cent outside these two limits. These figures do not necessarily point to natural very short (< 4 hours a night) or long sleepers (> 11 hours) who sleep like this every night, because these findings simply show the distribution over the whole 5,718 nights across all our volunteers—most of the short sleeping nights were when sleep was curtailed and the longer sleeps were lie-ins.

When the sleep quality of habitual five- and nine-hour sleepers is compared with the average sleeper with seven to seven and a half hours, then in terms of light, deep, and rapid eye movement (REM) sleep, the first five hours of sleep for all of the sleepers are virtually the same. The 'hypnogram' (Figure 13) illustrates this point, because both types of sleeper have similar amounts of deep (stages 3 and 4) sleep. In contrast, the short sleepers seem to have lost the last few hours of a longer sleep, which would have mostly consisted of light sleep (stages 1 and 2) and REM sleep. Figure 16 shows this important point another way, especially the remarkable consistency of deep sleep. It will be remembered, from Chapter 8, that, when long and short sleepers are sleep deprived for a night, long sleepers do not usually sleep for much longer than normal during the following recovery night, because this sleep seems to 'soak up' the essential parts of the lost sleep that has to be recovered, at the expense of light

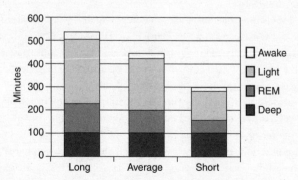

Figure 16 Habitual long, average, and short sleepers: differences in sleep structure.

sleep. This essential sleep is, of course, mostly deep sleep. Short sleepers, on the other hand, have to extend their recovery sleep to replenish lost deep sleep. It is as if they have no spare capacity within their normal sleep to absorb it. The average sleeper lies between these two extremes.

Very short sleepers

More extreme, healthy, naturally short (less than 4 hours of sleep a day) and long (more than 11 hours) sleepers, who sleep like this every night, are very rare but do exist. Both are fairly normal in the sense that the short sleeper is not a 'shortened' sleeper who used to sleep for longer and then decided to restrict him- or herself, nor does the longer sleeper have a sleep disorder. The key point is that both feel quite alert and are not dozing off during the waking day. Again, the four-hour sleepers have a very similar hypnogram to the first four hours of sleep for the rest of us. Healthy short and long sleepers do not differ much by way of intellect, and there is no support for the idea that short sleepers have a higher IQ or that long sleepers are dim. However, there is a tendency for short sleepers to be more gregarious and 'enthusiastic' people, which becomes even more apparent with the even rarer, extremely short sleeper who seems to survive very well on two to three hours sleep a day. They tend to be euphoric and even 'hypomanic'—with a mild but usually harmless type of mania.

In looking at natural short sleepers, usually sleeping about five hours a night (including weekends), Dr Tim Monk and colleagues,[2] from the University of Pittsburgh, found that these people had a more positive attitude to life and were more optimistic. Long sleepers, on the other hand, are more likely to be 'worriers', with a more depressive outlook on life. This is another illustration of the tantalising but not really understood link between sleep and mood, and it will be remembered that earlier I mentioned how severely depressed people could have their spirits raised when their sleep was severely restricted for one night—to four hours or less. However, this is an extreme instance, involving mentally ill people, and is unlikely to have much effect on the mood of the long but happy sleeper.

Whether or not very short sleepers remain healthy is something that remains to be clarified, although, later I will show some evidence to suggest that they may have a somewhat shorter life expectancy. The cynic might argue, of course, that life expectancy is not everything, because a somewhat shorter but happy life is more fulfilling than a longer, dreary existence.

We tend to credit great leaders with superhuman qualities and exaggerate their attributes, including their being able to survive on little sleep. Nevertheless, several famous leaders and notables were apparently short sleepers, such as Alexander the Great, Napoleon Bonaparte, and Thomas Edison. Interestingly, as all were somewhat hypomanic, this disposition can have its benefits and may well have helped to get them where they were. One co-worker said of Edison that, despite his being a short sleeper, 'his genius for sleep equalled his genius for invention. He could go to sleep anywhere, any time on anything'.[3] Always a night bird, Edison would often start work at dusk, have 'lunch' at midnight, and then go on until dawn. Believing that changing clothes was bad for creativity, he usually slept fully clothed. He claimed to sleep around four hours a night, and often catnapped in a cot at his office, although he was often found sleeping on the floor or on a nearby table. His sleeping at work nearly resulted in disaster, because he was fired from his first job, as a telegrapher, for not forwarding a message warning of a narrowly averted head-on train collision. Napoleon seems to have thrived on five or six hours of sleep a night, and was able to doze and wake at will. He would often wake up at midnight, go into his study, work for several hours, and then go back to bed.

Some years ago I met an elderly woman who seemed to sleep less than two hours a day. She was engaged in several ambitious projects including writing a book and painting numerous pictures. None of these works was ever completed, like the many others of her previously unfinished grand schemes. She talked to me almost continuously for what seemed like hours, and drank numerous cups of tea—about 20 a day by her reckoning. From what I saw and tasted, it was strong tea—and probably provided her with sufficient caffeine to keep her going, which must have been at least partly responsible for her short sleep. The point of this tale is that it is always a good idea to observe self-confessed very short sleepers before jumping to conclusions.

Although no healthy non-sleeper has ever been found, there are various unsubstantiated claims coming from newspapers that turn out to be bogus or gross distortions. Many self-claimed extremely short sleepers examined at sleep laboratories turn out to be people who are chronically sleep deprived, having forced themselves into taking little sleep. Others are, quite frankly, liars, out for the publicity. The majority, however, seem to be quite honest and are just grossly mistaken. For example, some people consider sleep to be only what occurs in bed with your pyjamas on, and dismiss the taking of naps in a chair as not being 'real sleep'. Other claimants genuinely do not realise when they have been asleep, and the true story comes to mind of a woman who professed not to sleep 'a wink' at night. She supported her claim by hearing a nearby church clock strike each hour. It turned out that, unbeknown to her, she regularly awoke throughout the night a few minutes before the hour (to hear the clock strike), returning to sleep a few minutes later!

Sadly, however, there is a very rare, inherited brain disease called, 'fatal familial insomnia', in which the brain slowly degenerates. In this tragic, hereditary illness, which begins with a loss of muscle control, sleep eventually disappears. Although sufferers often claim not to feel sleepy—maybe for many months initially, and apparently with little intellectual impairment—few careful assessments of their mental abilities have been described. At night, they commonly have dramatic hallucinations involving all the senses, and are often in much pain, especially in the hands and feet. These episodes last from 20 minutes to an hour, and seem to be dream like. However, because of the brain damage it is difficult to know if this is some form of aberrant sleep and, if so, whether the hallucinations are signs of REM sleep, as might be suspected. Sleeping tablets do not work, although treatment with other medicines that mimic the brain's own sleep substances can be effective for a while. Patients eventually go into an irreversible coma and die, usually within a year of the initial symptoms appearing. The extent to which their little or no sleep contributes towards death remains unknown.

More sleep

Most of us 'average' sleepers can easily take more sleep than our usual amount, but the question is 'Do we really need it?'. This is a hot topic for the next Chapter, but let me deal with one particular aspect, now. There have been many studies showing that, if volunteers are asked to continue lying in bed in the morning and not get up, they will happily sleep for an extra hour or two. We studied[4] this in healthy seven- to eight-hour sleepers without complaints of daytime sleepiness, who stayed in bed for ten hours overnight, for fourteen consecutive nights. During the rest of the day they carried on with their normal activities. Most found that they could easily sleep nine hours, but not for ten, and soon settled into this not unpleasant routine. To enable us to look for changes in daytime alertness, they were regularly tested with a prolonged and monotonous vigilance task where they had to listen out for a particular computer-generated 'beep' tone among an interminable series of longer 'beeeeeeps'. This was much more sensitive to sleepiness than the usual ten-minute reaction time test, and had to be lengthy so that we could eke out even the smallest sign of sleepiness. They also underwent the Multiple Sleep Latency Test (MSLT) during the daytime—a test of sleepiness measuring how long people take to fall asleep, which I will be coming to. To get to the point, the extra sleep had no effect on the vigilance task and the only benefit to the MSLT was that the afternoon 'dip' disappeared which might seem to be worthwhile, but, as we see, it was not really.

Although their night-time sleep increased, it took them longer to fall asleep and they were more likely to wake up during the latter part of sleep—it was as though their normal sleep had been stretched out to fill the extended period, with more waking 'cracks' appearing. After the fourteen days they had to revert back to their previously normal seven to eight hours of night-time sleep, which they were quite happy to do because most saw this ten hours in bed as wasteful. The only effect was a return of the afternoon dip, which was minor in most cases.

By the way, sleeping for an extra hour is one thing, but taking too much extra sleep, well and truly beyond one's usual morning awakening time, is likely to lead to 'post-sleep inertia' or the 'worn-out syndrome', lasting some hours and typified by lethargy, heavy limbs, difficulty getting going, and 'thick headedness'. It is a type of jetlag, because sleeping excessively when we do not usually do so confuses the body clock.

I mentioned at the beginning of this book that well-fed or confined animals sleep for longer than when in the wild, where they have to search for their dinner. The simple explanation is that confinement and safety lead to boredom, and so they just sleep more. Rather similar experiments were carried out on humans in a spate of studies around 30 years ago, which investigated the 'maximum capacity for sleep', whereby healthy people had to stay in bed and sleep as much as possible for one or two days continuously (apart from going to the toilet). This arrangement was different from the study just described, in that these volunteers had to sleep and sleep until they could sleep no more, even though they had already slept normally beforehand and were not sleep deprived. The findings were consistent in showing that most of them could sleep or doze for at least 12 hours during the first day, and some up to 15 hours. Much of this was fitful sleep, of course. The question was, and still is, 'Did they need it?'. I doubt it! Most of us eat and drink more than we need, certainly in excess of simply overcoming hunger and thirst. What about that extra helping of yummy dessert, all those cups of tea or coffee, or those tempting 'nibbles'? None is necessary, but merely a pleasant indulgence—so why not the same for sleep? Why can we not just have that sleep-in because we enjoy sleeping and want to be lazy, even though those weekend lie-ins might also be making up for some lost sleep from the previous weekdays?

Indeed, there are 'appetitive nappers',[5] who are able to nap even when not feeling sleepy, who can fall asleep almost anywhere if they so wish—typically mid-afternoon. Their night-time sleep is the same, irrespective of whether or not they take a daytime nap. Seemingly, they just enjoy napping!

Less sleep

Following a night or two without sleep, or even longer, and as shown by Drs Patrick and Gilbert, Randy Gardner (see Chapter 4), and many other sleep-deprived volunteers since then, only around a third to a half of the lost sleep seems to be reclaimed on recovery. Almost all of the lost deep sleep is recovered, with about half of the lost REM sleep, but most of the missing light sleep seems to be gone for good. In practical terms, someone who sleeps for seven and a half hours a night and loses all their sleep for a night, staying up until 9pm the next evening (when they probably cannot stay awake any more) will need to sleep about ten hours for a full recovery next morning, when he or she will wake up around the normal time. This sleep consists of the usual seven and a half hours, plus roughly a third of what was lost, with the total of ten hours containing double the usual amount of deep sleep.

Given a few weeks of gradual sleep reduction, people may well be able to adapt to taking less sleep, without increasing their day-time sleepiness. I am not advocating that we do so, especially for those people 'on the go' for much of the day, who obtain little rest during wakefulness. For them, sleep provides the only occasion for prolonged relaxation, and they should not be cutting down on their sleep, but probably taking more. Nevertheless, some sustained sleep reduction is possible, which was first shown in 1935, by Dr Richard Wellington Husband from the University of Wisconsin. It was not an ideal study because only one volunteer was recruited, introduced at the beginning of Husband's report as, 'Miss Helen Rose, a final year student, who offered to sacrifice herself physically and socially to carry out a fairly lengthy and rigid routine of sleep regulation' (p 792).[6] Initially she slept for one month at her normal eight hours a night, followed by another month sleeping six hours a night in two blocks of three hours each, separated by three hours of wakefulness from 2.00 to 5.00am. She spent this extra time 'writing, studying and sewing'. Each Saturday morning she was given a medical check-up and a battery of 11 tests that included: hand steadiness, finger tapping speed, card sorting, tracking, reaction time, a coding task, grip strength, body sway, and IQ measurement. Nothing of note was found, apart from what Husband described as 'suggestions as to very slight loss of efficiency in body sway and speed of tapping, but these were slight and inconsistent' (p 796).[6] However, he wisely observed that, for some tasks, the improvement with practice could have counteracted any detriment caused by sleepiness.

I mentioned the pitfalls of the 'practice effect' in Chapter 7. Unfortunately, this improvement with practice also leaves question marks over more recent sleep reduction studies, where volunteers systematically reduced their usual sleep from seven to eight hours per night, in steps of about half an hour, for a week each time, until they could go no further. Daytime naps were banned. The regimes lasted for several months, and throughout this period the participants kept sleep diaries, especially of the more tell-tale difficulties in getting up in the mornings and daytime sleepiness. Periodically, they would undergo the usual psychological tests, including reaction time, and had their sleep EEGs recorded at night. Although the tests showed little or no change over the study, a practice effect may well have crept in to counteract any decline, because there was no control group undergoing the same tests over the same period, who slept normally. Nevertheless, their diaries revealed that real problems did not start until around the five-hour level of sleep reduction, when they became irritable and showed obvious daytime sleepiness—clearly they had gone too far. As expected, sleep patterns showed that their restricted sleep was similar to their usual first five hours of sleep and, more to the point, without loss of deep sleep. Perhaps the most enlightening find was that eight months later, after they had been released from the study and were free to sleep as they wished, they were re-tested, and were found to be sleeping between six and six and a half hours a night. Seemingly, they had voluntarily reduced their old sleep length by at least an hour.

We carried out a similar study with healthy men and women in their mid-twenties, who normally slept about eight hours a night, and who promised to keep honest and accurate records of their sleep and daytime activities. Half of them were randomly put through the sleep restriction regime, described shortly, and the others slept normally, acting as a control group who did everything as did the reduction group, except for the restriction. The control group enabled us to assess any practice effects, which could be subtracted from the findings with the sleep reduction group, so that a net effect would largely be the result of the sleep reduction itself. It was also very important for us to have a good rapport with our volunteers because we just wanted to know the truth about whether and to what extent they could learn to reduce their daily sleep. There was no pressure on them to misrepresent sleep times and sleepiness ratings in their diaries. To encourage the reduced sleep regimen, alarm clocks had to be used every morning, but placed away from the bed to force them to get up to turn the alarm off! They avoided daytime naps and did not drink more than their usual amounts of tea and coffee. Alcohol intake had to be kept to a minimum.

After a week of familiarisation with various tests, the study began with an initial week of sleep restricted to an average of seven hours a night, followed by three weeks at six and a half hours a night, and finally two weeks at six hours of sleep. They could choose to do this by going to bed later, rising earlier, or doing some of both. The control group had to adhere to the exact bedtimes and arising times. Neither group was allowed days off, especially at weekends. All had regular psychological performance testing, especially at a lengthy reaction time test, as well as daytime EEG tests of sleepiness, similar to the MSLT. Periodically, they had overnight sleep EEGs recorded.

Sleep reduction was uneventful. No one pulled out, and all managed successfully to arrive at the sleep target of six hours. Although two experienced some difficulties waking up in the mornings, none reported any increased daytime sleepiness after the first few days of each reduction period. Over the weeks, both groups showed identical changes with all the tests of sleepiness. Indeed, there was a noticeable improvement and a clear practice effect, but similar for both groups. Night-time sleep for the reduction group showed little change to the first six hours of sleep, but they fell asleep more quickly and reported better sleep quality, with fewer awakenings—that is, sleep restriction improved their sleep quality. By the way, this type of sleep restriction can be useful in treating insomnia (see Chapter 20). I should add that restriction to six hours of sleep is just about the limit for most people, for both people with insomnia and normal sleepers alike.

There is a further twist to this tale, however. When we began this study, everyone, including the sleep reduction volunteers, thought that the extra wakefulness would allow more time for personal projects—but this was not to be. All that happened was that they used this extra time to waste time—a case of 'Parkinson's law', whereby the time taken for tasks simply expands to fit the time available! Maybe long sleepers are efficient people, able to do a day's work quickly and then have more time to sleep?

The ability to adjust our sleep length by an hour or so, gradually over time, makes sense when one considers how dependent on daylight and darkness humans used to be, until the comparatively recent appearance of artificial lighting. As we are so reliant on our eyes, and as our eyes need good light to see, we had little else to do in the dark except to sleep. Seasonal changes in daylight and darkness, becoming more profound the further one is away from the equator, would have encouraged us to adjust our sleep length according to the seasons—extending sleep during the winter to while away the long nights, and shortening it in the summer when there was a harvest to be gathered and daytime predators around. Provided that we feel fairly alert throughout the day, then, irrespective of its length, whatever sleep we have obtained at night is about right for us, and is probably a satisfactory and realistic compromise between being able to take a little more and being able to take a little less.

Leonardo da Vinci

Arguably, the best way of trying to cope with little sleep is not to take it in a single block each day, but under a 'little but often' regimen, perhaps in the form of 20-minute naps every 2 hours or so. This is feasible only under extreme conditions, and it takes at least a week or so of doing this before any benefits may be found. What is surprising is that, despite there being, at best, only about four hours of total sleep per day, sleepiness is much less than when the four hours of sleep is taken in a single, daily block. In fact, with this latter restriction, sleepiness becomes so overwhelming that a week of it is about the very limit. Anecdotally, the most famous exponent of the numerous 20-minute naps was Leonardo da Vinci, who would practise this method of sleeping for many weeks at a time, especially when painting huge wall murals. In those days, 500 years ago, the paint he used could not be allowed to dry for more than about 30 minutes, because it would crack when further paint was applied. So he had to keep on going until the masterpiece was finished. He coped surprisingly well on this routine, which is still used today, not by artists, but by solo yachtsmen and women in long distance races, who cannot take their eyes off their sails or the sea for more than a short while. Ellen MacArthur demonstrated this method, recently, in her record-breaking, solo, round-the-world venture, when she spent most of her 72 days at sea doing just this, with the occasional longer sleep taken in the days when she was becalmed.

Such 20-minute sleeps, taken within the context of chronic sleep loss, and after a week or so of adaptation, are more intense than the typical nap and contain more deep sleep than would otherwise be expected. These 'super-naps' are sufficient to allow for some worth-while recovery but are not so long a period as to lead to grogginess and confusion on awakening.

18 Are we chronically sleep deprived?

Irony

> The subject of sleeplessness is once more under public discussion. The hurry and excitement of modern life is held to be responsible for much of the insomnia of which we hear; and most of the articles and letters are full of good advice to live more quietly and of platitudes concerning the harmfulness of rush and worry. The pity of it is that so many people are unable to follow this good advice and are obliged to lead a life of anxiety and high tension.

So began the *British Medical Journal* editorial of 29 September 1894 (p 719).[1] All that needs to be done is to change the writing style a little to fit the modern idiom and the message is fit for today!

Increasingly, it is being claimed that seven to seven and a half hours of sleep per night, typical for many healthy adults, is insufficient, and that chronic sleep debt is becoming endemic in western populations. Seemingly, many of us are largely unaware of this apparent chronic sleepiness, and to avoid this state of affairs we should be taking up to nine hours of daily sleep. It is perhaps ironic that, whereas many physicians are prepared to believe a patient's self-diagnosis of insomnia, and then to prescribe treatment without any further assessment, a healthy person not complaining of sleepiness or inadequate sleep may have this opinion disregarded in favour of a chronic sleep debt and be professionally advised to take more sleep.

Much of the experimental evidence supporting this sleep debt is based on laboratory studies using 'gold standard' tests of sleepiness, similar to those mentioned in Chapter 7, particularly the Multiple Sleep Latency Test (MSLT), and reaction time tests. This is not criticism of these excellent tests, because they provide valuable contributions to our understanding of sleep, but I believe that they can all too easily lead to misleading interpretations in relation to the issue of 'sleep debt'. Moreover, over-generalisations from other findings, as well as ambiguity over the meaning of 'sleepiness', lead me to maintain that, nowadays, most adults do have adequate sleep, that any sleep debt, if evident, has not worsened in recent times, and this state of affairs has always been with us.

The sleep debt issue has wider implications, because advocating that we need more sleep may well cause further worry among people with insomnia, many of whom tend to be over-anxious about their health, anyway. Moreover, it may lead to unwarranted demands for sleeping tablets and other potions in people who, hitherto, have been reasonably content with seven or so hours of sleep a night. Sleep debt has also been linked to the 'metabolic syndrome', which can be seen as a mild, 'pre-diabetic' state whereby our bodies are less able to cope with sugar or carbohydrate intake. The disorder is largely associated with obesity, and I argue that rather than sleep beyond seven or so hours in an attempt to correct this syndrome, this extra time would be better spent in taking more exercise instead, especially as exercise is an established and effective treatment for dealing with it, as is reducing calorie intake.

Another misleading implication stemming from hidden sleep debt is that it might conceivably be produced as a medical problem, as an unjustifiable defence for sleep-related vehicle crashes. For example, 'my client thought they had adequate sleep, but in taking only seven hours sleep a night, it turns out that they have a chronic sleep debt, and was unaware of both it and the hidden sleepiness'.

This chapter looks at chronic sleep debt in relation to healthy adults who do not complain of chronic sleepiness, which, according to some schools of thought, is endemic in many western societies. However, I believe that much of this sleepiness is more imagined than real and, to a large extent, may well be an artefact of the laboratory setting.

Did we sleep for longer?

It is often proclaimed that the average sleep length for present-day adults has decreased from about nine hours per night, at the turn of the last century, to around seven hours today. This stems from the misinterpretation of research carried out 90 years ago[2] by Dr Lewis Terman and Miss Adeline Hocking, working at Stanford University, California. Although it is commonly assumed that their findings were based on sleep in adults, they did not study adult sleep at all, but that of some 2,000 8- to 17-year-old schoolchildren, assessed between 1910 and 1911. Given that this age group have always slept longer than adults anyway, it is unreasonable to compare them with today's adults. In their report, Terman and Hocking went on at length to explain that, 'the average child actually receives more sleep than he needs, that mind and body reach their highest efficiency with a definite, as yet minimum amount of sleep' (p 201). They even pointed out that the nine hours' average sleep in their young people (which seems reasonable, nowadays, for 8–17 year olds) was a 'striking excess of sleep', and about one hour longer than that reported by other findings at the time, from Germany, the UK, and Japan. By the way, also remarkable are the further accounts by Terman and Hocking of the long school hours for pupils in those days, with a reference to another study entitled, 'Overpressure in the Schools of Denmark', dated 1898, and based on 3,500 Danish schoolchildren, where it was noted that 'sleep was most deficient among pupils pursuing the arduous classical courses, where it often fell to 6 or 7 hours'!

Unfortunately, older historical accounts of how much sleep we adults used to take seem to be more anecdotal than factual. I mentioned in Chapter 5 how, 500 years ago, in Britain as well as throughout much of the rest of Europe, it was common to have an early evening sleep, called in old English '*fyrste slepe*' ('first sleep'). Typically, it was followed by supper, the main meal of the day attended by family and friends, or just in quiet contemplation, prayer, or pleasant thought. 'Second sleep', often called 'morning sleep', would usually not begin until the small hours. Hence, a continuous period of seven, eight, or even nine hours of sleep at night is probably a more recent western characteristic, maybe linked to industrialisation.

Perhaps one of the best known historical anecdotes about how much sleep we need, which is nowadays politically incorrect to mention, came from Napoleón Bonaparte, who exhorted, 200 years ago, 'six hours sleep for a man, seven for a woman and eight for a fool'. He certainly practised what he preached. But enough of these delicate matters—except to say that eight hours of sleep were generally regarded by the Victorians as a pleasure for the idle rich. For much of the working population in those days who, for six days a week, worked fourteen or even more hours a day, in addition to travelling to and from work, the opportunities for sleep were limited. Even on Sundays, the only regular day off, they would have to rise early and be obliged to go to church. For other contemporaries, sleep was even more of an ordeal, taken under the most uncomfortable of circumstances, because many of the Victorian poor, living in workhouses, never slept in a bed. Instead, they slept in lines sitting on benches, with their arms dangling over a taught rope, called a 'hangover', at chest height, that they literally hung over. How they slept like this is a mystery, but is a testament to the adaptability of people being able to sleep in the most awful of conditions. What is more, and to add to their misery, they would be charged for this privilege, by the hour, and the money deducted from their meagre wages.

Time in bed

'Sleep duration' or 'sleep need' can easily be seen to be synonymous with 'time in bed', and we have to be wary about what exactly people mean when they say how much sleep they need, and whether, for example, they see the latter as the time from 'lights out' to the end of fitful dozing in the morning, when they get out of bed. I suspect that popular claims that we need nine hours of sleep include this extra time in bed, spent going to sleep and waking up.

In the cold winters of not so long ago, impoverished people would spend many hours in bed simply to keep warm (a situation still found, today, among impecunious elderly people). Similarly, during economic recessions and in the great depression of the 1930s, whole families would stay in bed for days at a time, for the same reason—

which further illustrates that being in bed did not always equate with sleep or recovering from 'sleep debt'. Sleep was the least of their worries, as the bigger problem was food debt, or rather unemployment and starvation—if only they could complain of sleep debt! In some respects, sleep debt is the contemporary complaint for those of us who are well fed, well housed, and in full employment.

Support for the idea of a sleep-deprived contemporary society might come from our heavy reliance on alarm clocks, and that many of us do not feel alert immediately on getting up in the morning—with both signs indicating insufficient sleep. On the other hand, even the sleep-satisfied individuals among us still use an alarm clock to ensure punctuality. As for not being alert on arising, I have two answers: first, to my knowledge, no study allowing otherwise contented people to sleep in as long as they want has found any improvement in their alertness on eventually awakening in the morning. Second, we usually take some minutes to settle down after lights out at night, in the transition from awake to becoming sleepy and then falling asleep—so why can the reverse not be true for waking up in the morning, with some time needed before we are fully alert and ready to go?

Healthy sleep

Studies in the UK over the past 40 years,[3,4] including our own,[5] are consistent in showing that the average daily sleep for adults up to 70 years of age remains at about 7–7.5 hours. If one took the view that we need an hour or so more sleep, it seems that the British have been chronically sleep deprived for many years. On the other hand, a recent, very large American study by Dr Dan Kripke and colleagues from San Diego, involving over a million respondents, reported[6] that death rates were lowest in people sleeping around seven hours per day (which is about the average for the USA). His findings, seen below, showed that people sleeping beyond eight and a half hours had an increasing death rate. The same applied to those sleeping less than six hours a day, although this latter finding also seemed to be related to the increased use of sleeping tablets—that is, many of these shortened sleepers may have taken these tablets for night-time

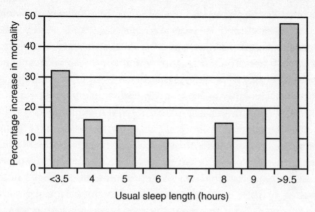

Figure 17 Mortality for different sleep lengths.

pain or other discomforts, and it is the latter that contributed towards death, not the sleeping tablets. Underlying factors affecting health, such as smoking, obesity, alcohol abuse, serious illnesses, and various medicines, were accounted for in Kripke's results (Figure 17).

Despite the shortcomings of his study (people were asked only one question about how long they slept), there are no other epidemiological data of similar size that can be utilised to argue differently. In fact, two more recent findings support him, as we shall see. Incidentally, if society has been chronically sleep deprived for so many years, and this causes ill-health, then it might be surprising that people are so much healthier and live longer nowadays than 100 years ago when daily sleep was supposedly much longer.

Of course, it would still be wise to treat Kripke's findings with caution, and foolish to claim that if the nine-hour sleepers reduced their sleep by an hour or so, and the six-hour sleepers increased their sleep by the same amount, both might enjoy longer lives. There are many reasons why people sleep longer or shorter than normal, and sleep length can simply be symptomatic of other underlying causes—for example, overwork and stress, which Kripke could not assess.

A good example of this comes from a Japanese study[7] that clearly

189

supported Kripke's conclusions. More than 100,000 men and women aged between 40 and 79 years were recruited from 1988 onwards, and their survival was monitored for almost 10 years, during which time 11,071 died. The respondents initially reported on their average sleep length during weekdays, their general health (including alcohol intake, smoking, exercise levels, education, marital status), as well as aspects of their mental health. From these findings, the average sleep length was 7 hours 29 minutes for men and 7 hours 7 minutes for women. Subsequently, the least deaths occurred among those who took seven hours of sleep, with mortality rising with increasing or decreasing sleep lengths—as with Kripke's findings. Interestingly, this later study also assessed overwork and stress in the respondents and, for the men, the higher mortality in the shorter sleepers disappeared when these two factors were taken into consideration—that is, stress and overwork may well have caused death and shortened sleep, rather than the shorter sleep causing death. A criticism of both these and Kripke's findings is that both relied on the participants providing self-reports of their sleep durations. However, if people did make mistakes over how much sleep they took, then there is no reason why these errors would have gone one way rather than another, and would have randomised out to make no difference.

The second study, by Dr Najib Ayas and colleagues[8,9] from Harvard Medical School, reported on the incidence of both coronary heart disease and 'late-onset diabetes' (these disorders are often related) in over 71,000 nurses during a 10-year period starting in 1986. In an initial questionnaire the nurses provided information on their usual daily sleep. Subsequently, those sleeping between six and a half and seven and a half hours per day had a nine per cent increased risk of heart disease compared with those who slept between seven and a half and eight and a half hours. Other potential health hazards such as smoking and obesity were accounted for. Those having around 6 hours, or over 9 hours, of sleep had 18 per cent and 38 per cent more risk, respectively, whereas those who slept less than 5 hours had 45 per cent more risk. For diabetes, the findings were slightly different, as those sleeping between 6.5 and 8.5 hours had a low risk for this disease, whereas for others sleeping around 6 hours it was 13 per cent greater, and for those sleeping less than 5 or over 9 hours it was around 37 per cent greater.

Although this study might suggest that nine hours sleep is inadvisable, that around seven hours is not the most ideal after all, and that eight hours is better, it must be remembered that nurses do tend to lead disrupted lifestyles, which affects sleep. Thus, judging their sleep solely by its length provides only one perspective on this complex issue, and the relatively small, nine per cent extra risk of heart disease (but not for diabetes) for the six-and-a-half- to seven-and-a-half-hour sleepers must be judged accordingly. The findings with diabetes are particularly interesting, because I have already mentioned that short sleep, even seven hours, might be thought to be a risk factor for this illness. But this is not supported, here, although both six and nine hours of sleep may well present greater risks in this respect.

Just over seven hours a night is the average sleep duration when rapid eye movement (REM) sleep becomes much more intense, as shown by particularly intense rapid eye movements during REM sleep—a finding that led the investigator, Eugine Aserinsky[10] (the co-discoverer of REM sleep—see Chapter 14), to conclude that this is the point of sleep satiety, when 'some physiological function had approached saturation as a result of sleep' (p 153). Subsequent research[11] supports his views and, for example, MSLT findings show that when night sleep exceeds seven and a half hours, the further improvement in daytime alertness is fairly small, although it does pick up somewhat as sleep increases to nine and a half hours. Nevertheless, the cost-effectiveness of such a long sleep must be doubtful, and around seven hours of sleep at night is a satisfactory compromise for most people, reflecting prudence rather than chronic sleep debt.

Other claims that people sleep less nowadays, compared with many years ago are also debatable when the evidence is scrutinised. Another study[12] from the USA was based on a mental health survey of over 500 healthy men and women, archived since the 1930s. An identical survey was again undertaken in the 1990s, recruiting a similar number of healthy people from the same geographical area. Among all the questions asked (with most having no relevance to sleep) there were two clusters relating to 'disturbed sleep' and 'daytime fatigue' respectively. It was found that there was no difference between the groups for disturbed sleep. Apart from for daytime fatigue, fewer of the recent respondents claimed to feel 'rested' or 'energetic', and more had 'trouble functioning' or less 'stamina' (these were the exact terms used). However, this applied only to the men, because the women did not differ over this 60-year gap in time. The extent to which feeling less 'rested' or 'energetic', etc, is synonymous with daytime sleepiness and insufficient sleep is anyone's guess, especially as perhaps the most appropriate descriptor for daytime fatigue—relating to the question 'Do you nap in the day?'—produced no differences for either men or women over this 60-year period. I return to the interpretations of 'sleepiness', 'fatigue', 'tiredness', and other synonyms later. Suffice it to say that the only clear conclusion that one can draw from the meanings of these words is that they convey different things to different people.

Restricting sleep in healthy adults to four hours a day, for six days, leads[13] to symptoms of the 'pre-diabetic metabolic syndrome', mentioned earlier. Technically it means 'impaired glucose tolerance due to increased insulin resistance'. From this one could easily conclude that insufficient sleep alone, indeed produces physical illness, without there being other stresses, such as overwork and 'burning the candle at both ends', that can certainly lead to illnesses as well as cause sleep loss. It should be remembered that more severe, total sleep loss studies in both humans and rats (see Chapter 3) found little to this effect. On the other hand, and to be fair, this recent finding relating to the metabolic syndrome might fit in with those nurses[9] who slept less than five hours a night and seemed to have a higher incidence of diabetes.

Volunteers for this four-hour sleep restriction experiment were confined to bed (apart from going to the toilet) during the last two days, so that measurements could be made more easily. Four hours of sleep per day is very difficult to maintain for more than a few days, as we ourselves have discovered from our own work. Beyond about four days of this regimen people become extremely sleepy and cannot stay awake without intervention to prevent sleep, even when they are sitting—when lying awake it is impossible. Even the investigators noted that their volunteers became very sleepy, and it is possible that in struggling to stay awake they found the situation stressful. Indeed, a significant rise in levels of the stress hormone cortisol (see Chapter 1) was reported. Unfortunately, the real extent of this potential additional stress was unable to be measured, which is a pity, because another study[14] has noted that the psychological effect of anticipating a shortened sleep, even for one night, leads to a marked rise in the closely related hormone (adrenocorticotrophin) an hour or so before being awoken. By the way, as soon as those four-hour, sleep-restricted volunteers were allowed their recovery sleep, the metabolic syndrome disappeared.

This study has important implications, and we must avoid overstating its conclusions—for example, that the 'pre-diabetic state' found might also be evident in people sleeping six or even seven hours. More worryingly, it might be concluded that the outcome from this study portends unfortunate consequences of sleep debt for society at large. To place all this on a more realistic footing, however, four hours of sleep per night for several nights is far too little sleep, likely to be stressful, and certainly abnormal to the extent that the outcome is perhaps not surprising. Few people attempt to, or indeed can, survive on such a low amount of daily sleep.

Hidden sleepiness?

Support for the idea that many people are chronically sleep deprived stems from using very sensitive tests of sleepiness, such as the MSLT, and I would like to look at this test and these findings in more depth. The MSLT requires participants to retire to a quiet and dimly lit bedroom, lie down, and be instructed to 'relax, close your eyes and try and go to sleep'. They remain like this for up to 20 minutes, or until the onset of light sleep, whichever is the sooner. The session is ended and the time to fall asleep ('sleep latency') from the beginning of the test is noted. The procedure is repeated every two hours, usually from 10am until 4 or 6pm, and the four or five sleep latency values are averaged to give the overall 'MSLT score'. Values between 10 and 15 minutes are seen to reflect 'mild' daytime sleepiness, 5–10 minutes as 'moderate', and below 5 minutes as 'severe' sleepiness.

However, normal, healthy people, without self-reported daytime sleepiness or sleep complaints can have MSLT scores under

10 minutes and one might conclude that they must suffer from chronic sleep loss, even if there is no other proof of their being sleepy. It can all too easily lead to the conclusion that these putative sufferers are simply unaware of their sleepiness, because it is a chronic condition and they have forgotten what real alertness feels like. Fair enough, but without corroboration this assumption has to be questioned.

Inasmuch as many apparently, but unknowingly, sleepy people can also easily extend their night-time sleep, this would seem to add further support to any claim that they are actually sleepy and sleep deprived. However, most do not feel the need to take regular daytime naps, which would be a sign of insufficient sleep. Although extending a night's sleep would improve (that is, lengthen) their MSLT scores, this usually averages only two to three minutes, with the main effect confined to the afternoon measurement session. A few minutes may be statistically significant, but it is not very much, especially as, outside this afternoon dip, these people, having had that extra sleep at night do not feel much more alert over the rest of the day. Moreover, the extra sleep is unlikely to improve their reaction times by very much. So, the alternative answer to all this is that they can just fall asleep easily during the MSLT, without being particularly sleepy—that is, during the day they are simply very good at going to sleep whenever they want to or, alternatively, they can quite easily stay awake and remain normally alert—whatever they choose.

A difficulty with the MSLT in relation to normal sleepers and the sleep debt issue is that testing covers only a third to a half of the usual waking day, usually between 10am and either 4 or 6pm as I just mentioned. Given that people also judge daily sleepiness by when they start to feel sleepy in the evening and whether they need an 'early night', the rather early ending of the MSLT misses this potentially important part of the day. Moreover, as most of the people used in these studies are young adults, they are more likely to be 'owls', whose wakefulness beyond the end of the MSLT sessions may take on greater relevance.

The typical setting for the MSLT comprises a sleep laboratory, a quiet, comfortable, and dimly lit bedroom, with the participant lying on a bed and encouraged to fall asleep—that is, there is a high expectancy by everyone, especially the participant, to nod off. Parallels can be drawn in assessing hunger between meals. When asked if they are hungry, most satiated healthy people in a situation not suggestive of eating will truthfully deny this. But sit them in a restaurant and present them with a menu and the opportunity for a free meal, then many will select from the menu and willingly consume what is served up. Were they hungry after all and experiencing a hidden food debt?

The MSLT is an excellent test in the right circumstances, but in relation to hidden sleep debt findings can be misleading. For example, simply altering one's sleeping position can have a large effect on the outcome of this test. Reclining in a comfortable chair rather than lying down can increase MSLT scores by 50 per cent[15]—even changing the number of pillows can influence matters. Obviously, all this contravenes the rules of the MSLT procedure, and so the thresholds for 'mild' and 'moderate' sleepiness would have to be adjusted. Nevertheless, it is unwise to designate people as suffering from chronic sleep debt simply on the basis of the MSLT, which is so sensitive to other factors. This is further reflected in what people do just before they undergo the MSLT sessions—even simple acts such as walking versus watching TV will affect the outcome. Giving monotonous psychological tests beforehand will almost certainly cause people to fall asleep faster during a subsequent MSLT. On the other hand, and in defence of the MSLT, it might be contested that all that happens, here, is for the boring task to relax people to their true level of sleepiness and, to use the technical term, their sleepiness is 'unmasked'. Or, is it like sitting contented and satiated in that restaurant, when someone comes along with another helping of that mouth-watering banoffi pie, and you eat it? Was a tiny, remaining sensation of hunger unmasked, or was it maybe pure self-indulgence?

What about those ever-dozing but confined zoo animals, who would otherwise be more alert and running around in the wild? Their sleepiness is affected by their surroundings, so why not the same for us? In one of my own experiments we found that when healthy, non-sleep-deprived people undergoing the MSLT were unexpectedly told that they will receive money for falling asleep as soon as possible, they would snuggle down more readily, fluff up their pillows with renewed interest, and fall asleep faster, especially during the afternoon—which can make the difference as to whether they were classed as mildly or moderately sleepy.

Supersensitivity?

Sleepy people characteristically show lapses or maybe microsleeps during dull and monotonous tasks. Between lapses, responses are usually close to normal. The monotony and boredom of these tests are worsened when one is all-too familiar with the task and it is well practised beforehand. Good laboratory procedures require that the experimental setting be uninterrupted by noise and other distractions, with participants seated alone in a sound-proofed, dimly lit, and visually sterile setting, so that they can attend fully to the test. Healthy people allowed up to eight hours of sleep a night still show lapses under repeated testing in these conditions, with lapses becoming steadily worse over successive days—all too easily blamed on sleep debt. Moreover, as participants are often oblivious to their poor performance under these circumstances and deny sleepiness, this again could be attributed to their not knowing that they were sleepy.

Another explanation for this poor performance is linked to the unrelenting monotony of the testing situation, including the waiting before being tested. In another study of ours,[16] we asked alert, non-sleep-deprived people to wait alone in a lounge for half an hour before ten minutes of reaction time testing, also under the usual rigorous and sterile conditions just described. We wanted to see what the effect of boredom during the waiting period would have on the test. In one condition, the waiting area contained dreary and outdated magazines on farm machinery, with the TV showing a tedious video of how to grade potatoes. In the other, there were topical magazines and an exciting sports video to watch. Subsequently, there were more lapses during the reaction time test following the dull wait.

Under similar testing conditions, healthy sleepers who do not complain of sleepiness are not necessarily sleepy, despite showing lapses, because these might not be caused by 'microsleeps'. To stay awake or avoid tedium, sleepy or bored people seek stimulation. Even in the sterile settings of these performance tasks it is likely that they will search for or even manufacture some form of stimulation, which distracts them from the task in hand, especially when the test is being repeated endlessly. They might start staring at cracks in the ceiling, create imaginary pictures from marks on the wall, or make words out of the first line of letters on the computer keyboard. In doing so they can miss the stimulus appearing on the screen—and there is your lapse! So, it is possible that some of these lapses attributed to sleepiness are not droopy-eyed microsleeps, but just distractions. Of course, it could be argued that a distraction is a sign of sleepiness, anyway, and it does not really matter whether a lapse is a microsleep or a distraction, because both result from sleepiness. Even if true, I argue that such a distraction results from a lesser degree of sleepiness than evident in a microsleep. By assuming that all lapses are microsleeps it might be concluded that participants in these studies are more sleepy than might be the case, whereas they are only fighting off endless drudgery and desperate for something different. Regrettably, as everything is now computerised, we know little about what participants really do in these situations.

Self-insight

Implicit within the chronic sleep debt idea is that there is some sleepiness of which we are unaware. As already mentioned, it may well be that we have been in this state for so long that we have forgotten what it is like to be more alert. This is why these more objective tests such as the MSLT and reaction time tests can flush it out. Yet, for this sleepiness to materialise, people doing these tests have to be lying down or sitting under boring conditions for at least five minutes before any sign of sleepiness is detected. Put differently, even the very best of these tests cannot detect sleepiness immediately, and to assume that they are better than our own self-insight is unreasonable unless we, too, have been lying or sitting relaxed for a comparable amount of time, before thinking about how sleepy we are. Often, participants in these studies only have a minute in which to complete a self-rating scale of their sleepiness, before being ushered into the more sustained experimental settings of the MSLT or reaction time measurement. Until fair comparisons are made to show otherwise, I argue that healthy sleepers (excluding those with chronic, serious sleep disorders who indeed may have forgotten what it feels like to be alert) do have a good insight into their sleepiness.

Sleepability

If healthy, fully sleep-satisfied people with exactly the same sleep lengths have their sleep reduced by two hours for one night, then some will have shorter MSLT scores than others, despite the same sleep loss—that is, for any fixed amount of sleep loss there is a natural human variation (a 'normal distribution') in the ability to fall asleep. Is it because they do indeed differ in sleepiness despite having identical levels of sleep and sleep restriction? Or, do they have identical levels of sleepiness, with some easily falling asleep and others having more difficulty in doing so? We have found[17] people with no complaint of daytime sleepiness, having normal night-time sleep, and with low MSLT scores (indicative of moderate sleepiness), who then extended their sleep for several hours but still showed no change to the MSLT. Maybe they had a subtle sleep problem that was not easy to spot? Yet, when we initially gave them a very lengthy (one hour), exceedingly monotonous reaction time test, before that extra sleep, they performed equally as well as those people with normal MSLT scores. It seems that these particular people can fall asleep easily if they so wish, or just stay awake like any other normally alert person. I have called this 'sleepability without sleepiness'. Another example were those 'appetitive nappers' I mentioned earlier, who are able to nap wherever they wish, without feeling any particular need for sleep.

Separation of 'sleepability' from sleepiness also seems appropriate for people who have been treated for the complaint of 'obstructive sleep apnoea' (see Chapter 21), who, before treatment had severe daytime sleepiness and were, embarrassingly, always falling asleep. When successfully treated to remove the apnoea and the sleepiness, so that they could feel alert and no longer liable to drop off spontaneously, many still found that they could fall asleep quickly, *but only if they wished to do so*. I emphasise those last eight words, because this happens when they undergo the MSLT, after having been told to 'relax, shut your eyes, and go to sleep'. They fall asleep rapidly, and it gives the appearance that treatment has failed—and that they are still sleepy. Fortunately, most are much more alert than this and know it! The answer, it seems, is that all those years of suffering made falling asleep both easy and rapid—an ability that endures even with low levels of sleepiness after successful treatment. But the difference, now, is that they can easily decide whether or not to sleep, and effortlessly override falling asleep if they do not want to—that is, they have high sleepability with little or no sleepiness. Again, this means that not everyone having low MSLT scores, but without any complaint of sleepiness, is necessarily sleepy from chronic sleep debt.

Separation of sleepiness from sleepability is further indicated by the medicine, modafinil (marketed as Provigil®). It is a stimulant-like drug used not only for treating people with excessive sleepiness caused by serious sleep disorders, especially 'narcolepsy' (see Chapter 15), but also in military-type operations to knock out sleepiness and keep people awake. Despite little sleepiness after having taken this medicine, people can still go to sleep if they wish to, which contrasts with real stimulants, such as caffeine, which also prevent sleep. It is as though modafinil allows sleepability without much sleepiness.

The dip

Humans are designed to have two sleeps per day—the main one at night and a smaller one in the early to mid-afternoon. In warmer climates throughout the world, where it is particularly hot at this time, it is usual to have a 'siesta' (derived from the Latin *sexta hora*—sixth hour [after awakening]). Noel Coward, the playwright and singer, probably explained it all in his famous but now rather politically incorrect song, 'Mad dogs and Englishmen', which opens with:

> In tropical climes there are certain times of day
> When all the citizens retire,
> to tear their clothes off and perspire.
> It's one of those rules that the biggest fools obey,
> Because the sun is much too sultry and one must avoid
> its ultry-violet ray—

> The locals grieve when the English leave their huts,
> Because they're obviously, absolutely nuts.
> Only mad dogs and Englishmen go out in the midday sun.

Put more stuffily, humans originally evolved from equatorial areas where it was pointless to do anything but rest when the sun was overhead. Moreover, as our predators were similarly indisposed by the heat, why not use this period to reduce the more lengthy night sleep when those predators are about? For people living in hot climates, the siesta can last for up to two hours. Even in colder, more northern and southern latitudes, and among those of us who do not siesta, we still tend to have an afternoon propensity to sleep, but it is mostly a vestige—just a dip, when the afternoon MSLT sessions have their shortest sleep latencies. Nevertheless, it is natural and, within, limits, not indicative of sleep loss unless there has been a poor night's sleep, when the dip becomes much more obvious. One notable exception of someone living in colder climates, who invariably took full-blown afternoon siestas, was Winston Churchill:[18]

> You must sleep sometime between lunch and dinner, and no half-way measures. Take off your clothes and get into bed. That's what I always do. Don't think you will be doing less work because you sleep during the day. That's a foolish notion held by people who have no imagination. You will be able to accomplish more. You get two days in one—well, at least one and a half, I'm sure. When the war started, I *had* to sleep during the day because that was the only way I could cope with my responsibilities.

Not only would he sit up in bed after his siesta and happily dictate letters to his secretaries, in his pyjamas, but as a result of this siesta he needed only about four hours of sleep at night, and did not go to bed until very late. It meant that his staff had to work what seemed to them to be very arduous shifts.

Back to more mundane matters! Given that the most obvious outcome from extending one's normal night-time sleep by an hour or so is the elimination of the afternoon dip, wherein the main effect on the MSLT lies, it might be argued that we do need this extra hour's sleep after all. On the other hand, by assuming that a moderate afternoon dip is normal, this extra night-time sleep should not be viewed as lost sleep within the context of sleep debt, but, rather, as extra or 'super-normal' ('supersaturated') night sleep—in which case, absence of the afternoon dip is not the norm and not something to be sought after. Let me explain a bit more clearly. Extra morning sleep can be likened to an extra large breakfast sufficient to eliminate hunger at lunchtime, as well as the need for lunch itself. Such inefficient dietary management will also mean that the extra food consumed at breakfast, to alleviate lunch, will be greater than the food usually eaten for lunch. Best, then, to stick with a normal breakfast and lunch. Similarly, if we have a chronic sleep debt, it might not be so large as to need an hour or two more sleep at night, but better rectified by a more timely, efficient, and much shorter afternoon nap lasting maybe only 15 minutes. This would seem to be our natural state of affairs and would help our ancestors to avoid sleeping beyond sunrise when there was work to be done!

Finally, a brief return to coffee, or rather to claims that increased caffeine consumption in recent times is another sign of sleep debt, particularly to counteract that afternoon dip. Maybe we just enjoy the taste of coffee and caffeinated drinks! Besides, if sleep debt were to blame for this coffee consumption, it would be difficult to see why we also like coffee-tasting ice-cream and coffee icing on doughnuts, cakes, and cookies—not for the caffeine, surely?

Semantics

A fascinating study[19] on the sleep of over 12,000 Finnish people aged 33–60 years found that 20 per cent complained of insufficient sleep, with most of the latter claiming to sleep less than seven hours a night, but believing that they ought to be sleeping over nine hours. Nine years later, on follow-up, almost half (44 per cent) of these latter people were still of the same opinion. Given that each may have endured over 6,000 hours of lost sleep over those 9 years (that is, 9 years × 365 days × 2 hours per night), we might wonder how they survived. I am not being facetious over what is a matter of concern for these people, but clearly something is not right here. Clues come from further findings with this investigation, because the respondents also complained of stressful lives, long work hours, poor life satisfaction, and signs of depression—that is, although the original survey focused on insufficient sleep, this was probably not the real problem; more likely, it was the desire of these people to have more 'time out', with extra sleep being one way of achieving it. Simply giving them another hour or so of daily sleep is unlikely to be the real solution.

Other, similar studies have found that satisfaction with one's sleep is not necessarily associated with sleep itself, but the feeling of well-being, to the extent that people dissatisfied with their sleep may not be made happier simply by focusing on sleep improvement, which is a maxim applying to many people with insomnia, as we see in Chapter 19.

Just now I mentioned that terms such as 'daytime fatigue', 'feeling rested', 'trouble functioning', 'stamina', and 'energetic' could (but perhaps wrongly) be seen to be synonyms or antonyms of sleepiness, particularly in the context of chronic sleep debt. Perhaps the most commonly used synonym for 'sleepy' is 'tired', and I would like to concentrate on this word for a while, because many people, on hearing that someone was tired, would assume that they were needing sleep. However, 'tired' has a much wider use in the English/American lexicon than 'sleepy' does.

In the course of the development of arguably the best-known self-rating scale of mood, known as the 'Profile of Mood States' (POMS),[20] the authors reported differences in how people interpreted 'tired' and 'sleepy'. For example, whereas tired was linked to the feelings of being tense, anxious, and depressed, sleepy was seen to have the opposite connotation—of being relaxed. Moreover, sleepy, unlike tired, was also linked to 'confused'. As a result of these ambiguities these authors abandoned both 'sleepy' and 'tired' and, instead, resorted to the word 'fatigue', because people had a clearer view of what that meant—worn out, listless, exhausted, sluggish, weary, or bushed. My point is that just because someone says that they are tired (or, indeed, sleepy), we should not assume that they need sleep.

Even a widely used self-rating scale of sleepiness, the Stanford Sleepiness Scale (SSS),[21] contains some ambiguous words and phrases such as: 'able to concentrate', 'a little foggy', 'not at peak', 'let down', 'fogginess', 'slowed down', 'woozy', 'able to think clearly', and 'prefer to be lying down'. Again, these are not necessarily synonyms or antonyms of 'sleepiness'. For example, many people find that, when they extend sleep in the morning and sleep to capacity, to the level that they feel groggy on awakening with 'post-sleep inertia', they are unlikely to take even more sleep. Nevertheless, they may appear even more sleepy, because the grogginess makes them respond positively to many of the terms just mentioned, which are not real descriptors of sleepiness. This is why unambiguous scales for self-rated sleepiness must be used, similar to the one given in Chapter 7.

On a lighter note, faded paintwork and a limp lettuce can be described as 'tired', but not 'sleepy', and one can become 'tired' of that dreadful, long-running TV show. Even the Microsoft Word® thesaurus on my computer provides twice as many synonyms for 'tired' compared with 'sleepy'. Simply, then, 'tiredness' is not only indicative of insufficient sleep.

Plus ça change

Let me summarise this rather lengthy chapter. Healthy adults who sleep for around seven hours a night may experience a contentious area of sleepiness, best described as, 'some sleepiness which I do not really notice unless I lie down and relax for a while—which is mostly evident in the afternoon'. It might be seen to reflect a need for more sleep, whereas I argue that this is the normal 'human condition', consisting of a minor amount of sleepiness, within the bounds of normality, and acceptable to most of us. There is nothing to show that eliminating this sleepiness by increasing our daily sleep to nine hours, for example, will have any benefit for the high-level thinking skills described in Chapter 8, such as critical reasoning and IQ performance, as well as 'executive' functions such as decision-making, linguistic ability, most aspects of memory, insight, and being innovative and creative. Thus, the basis for taking more sleep in order to alleviate a subjectively unnoticed sleep debt is really discernible only by using the sophisticated facilities of a sleep laboratory and needs more substantiation. If need be, why not just have a short afternoon nap, or even drink a moderate amount of coffee (caffeine) to remove that modest level of daytime sleepiness, as indeed most healthy people do, and seemingly to no ill-effect?

Confined animals clearly have the ability to sleep longer than in the wild, so why should the same not apply to us, if the circumstances allow? We can eat and drink for pleasure rather than for any physiological need, so why not the same for sleep? The idea, for example, that on weekdays (that is, work days) we obtain inadequate sleep, resulting in a sleep debt, which is the reason for a 'lie-in' over the weekend, to pay off this debt, may be true in some respects. But it ignores the idea that a lie-in is also just for pleasure. If those people who endure some sleep restriction during weekdays continue to do so through the weekend, there is evidence that they may adapt to this, within reason. The weekend lie-in may simply destroy this potential adaptation, and one is 'back to square one' on Monday. Of course, I do not advocate such sleep restriction regimes, because I enjoy my sleep. However, such regimes can produce a more rapid falling asleep after 'lights out', and better sleep quality, with fewer interim awakenings—which is a technique that can be helpful to people with insomnia (see Chapter 20).

If people are asked directly if they would like more sleep, most say 'yes', in the same way they say 'yes' to, 'would you like: a higher salary, longer vacations, more time with your family, etc', which biases the result. We[22] looked at the 'need' for more sleep in over 10,000 adults, using a questionnaire that avoided this leading question and determined sleep shortfalls indirectly. Shortfalls were probed in two ways, by asking people how sleepy they were in the daytime (using the scale on page 238), and asking those who seemed to want more sleep, 'if you had an extra hour in the day, how would you spend it? Attractive choices included: reading, socialising, watching TV, exercise, and sleeping. For those seeming to want more sleep, the extent of this bore no relationship with daytime sleepiness, and only 20% of them opted for 'sleep', when given the alternatives. Again, it seems that 'more sleep' belies different needs and meanings.

Some years ago I proposed that the first part of sleep, wherein most of our deep sleep lies, is a particularly important form of sleep (for cortical recovery), which I called (and still do), 'core' sleep. As the pressure for sleep declines over the night, sleep is further maintained by what I then called 'optional' sleep, which is fairly adaptable and allows for some lengthening or shortening of total sleep time. I was wrong, then, in assuming that this optional sleep was as low as five hours of sleep, because not even I can survive on this amount. I need six hours at least, feel better with six and a half hours and best with around seven hours. Furthermore, I should have called this latter part of sleep 'adaptable' sleep or even 'flexi-sleep', because 'optional' conveys a rather flippant 'take it or leave it' type of sleep, when in fact it takes some time to adapt to modest sleep restrictions. On the other hand, nine hours of sleep is beyond the needs of most healthy adults and, historically, it always has been, even though most of us can increase our daily sleep to this extent given the opportunity and, more importantly, the incentive to do so. Around seven hours or so of uninterrupted, quality sleep at night is quite satisfactory for most healthy adults, maybe helped by the addition of a timely and short (for example, 15 minutes) afternoon nap.

Rather than assume that more sleep will improve health, we should weigh this up against the greater benefit that would probably be gained through utilising this extra time for taking more exercise instead. Exercise is a tried and tested anodyne for many of the ills of contemporary society, such as those associated with obesity, heart disease, and diabetes, and contrasts with any assumption that more sleep will help combat these disorders. It also points to the need for a much wider cost-versus-benefit analysis of us striving for a society devoid of any daytime sleepiness.

Well over 100 years have elapsed since those wise words in that *British Medical Journal* editorial. Indeed, 'the topic of sleepiness is once more under public discussion', and the 'hurry and excitement of modern life' is just as much a part of human nature and our continuing desire for progress. 'Much of the insomnia of which we hear' is still because we 'ignore the exhortations to live more quietly and avoid rush and worry' (p 719).[1] To be sure, the pity of it all remains 'that so many people are unable to follow this good advice and are obliged to lead a life of anxiety and high tension'. Thus, our sleeping life has not really changed and, if anything, is better today than for the average worker 100 or so years ago, who would have been most fortunate in having a comfortable bed of their own, in a warm and safe abode. In another 100 years we will probably be sleeping much the same as we do now, when another sleep researcher may once more find that *British Medical Journal* editorial[1] and muse: 'How little times have changed.'

19 Things that go bump in the night

Sleeplessness

During our study[1] of people's sleep at home, described in Chapter 12, the participants were asked to note down what caused them to wake up at night, if they happened to do so. Just over 6,400 reports were logged, which works out to about once a night per person. Estimates, next morning, of how long the awakenings lasted were mostly between five and ten minutes. The number and duration did not differ much between the sexes, or with increasing age, but there were important differences in the causes, as shown shortly. For 70 per cent of the awakenings the reports were that it was easy to get back to sleep afterwards, whereas for 23 per cent it was 'with difficulty', and for the remaining 7 per cent 'very difficult', where 'worry' was the main reason. Overall, the most common explanations tended to be 'don't know' or 'woke up thinking about something'.

I will describe the outcome for the 50–70 year olds separately from the two younger groups (aged 20–35 and 36–49 years), which I am combining because of their similarity (Figure 18). For those aged 20–49 years, there was a huge sex difference in the main causes of awakenings, because 'children' was the most likely reason for women. Not remarkable perhaps, but what was surprising, considering our enlightened age for equality of the sexes, was that so few men were woken up by their kids. For every five occasions that mum was woken up in this way, dad woke up only once! To add to the irony, women were more than twice as likely to be woken up by their bed partner than men. Overall, and largely for these two reasons, the women were almost twice as likely to be awoken. For the men the most commonly

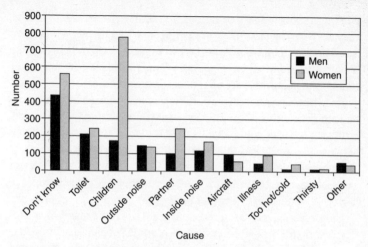

Figure 18 Causes of 3,837 awakenings in 20–49 year olds.

reported reason for their awakening, apart from 'don't know', was 'toilet'.

For the 50–70 year olds, women woke up half as much again as did the men and, for both, the most common reason was 'toilet' (Figure 19). Interestingly, these women were particularly sensitive to noise,

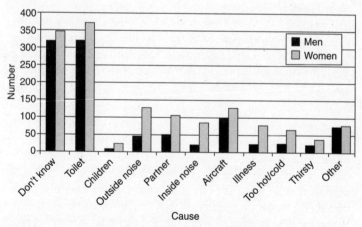

Figure 19 Causes of 2,585 awakenings in 50–70 year olds.

whether it was indoors or outdoors and, like the younger women, they were still twice as likely as men to be woken up by their partner. Also, older women were about five times more likely to be woken up by aircraft noise than were younger women, whereas this was three times more likely for older men than for younger men.

Remember, we excluded all those people who were often awoken by pain of one sort or another, or were taking sleeping tablets, especially as the latter could give us the false impression that sleep was better than it really was. All this resulted in the exclusion of about six per cent of all our potential volunteers. For those excluded, the main cause of pain was arthritis for the oldest people, whereas it was low back pain of one sort or another for the younger ones.

Undoubtedly, mental stress, strains, and worry are major causes for sleepless nights and, even during sleep, some people carry on worrying. It can lead to a form of tense, unrefreshing sleep, often associated with a type of low and middle-back pain called 'fibromyalgia', most apparent on arising. There seems to be no physical cause and it is not caused by rheumatism or a slipped disc, for example. Sufferers are often 'tired' but not particularly sleepy during the day. Our own studies of this disorder indicated that sufferers spend an unusual amount of time 'ruminating' in their sleep. Exactly what they ruminate about is unclear, but it seems to be a persistent agitation or worry at the 'back of one's mind'. Needless to say, one way or another, sufferers may be quite miserable as well, even a little depressed. Sometimes, help with fibromyalgia can come with tackling the stress and worries, through counselling, relaxation techniques, and perhaps some use of muscle relaxant medicines. Fibromyalgia can also be a symptom of a more severe form of 'tired all the time' insomnia, which is dealt with shortly.

The Victorians

Now for a lighter note! The nineteenth century burgeoned with inventions and ideas. Insomnia was probably as much of a problem then as it is now. Aids to better sleep abounded as did notions about what sleep was for. Some thought that it was caused by 'brain congestion' from blood accumulating in the head, whereas others advocated the exact opposite—a 'cerebral anaemia' caused by blood being withdrawn from the brain to aid digestive processes. Such contrasting ideas soon led to opposing beliefs about how to get 'better' sleep. On the one hand, the 'congestors' proposed sleeping with pillows under the feet—to encourage blood to the head—whereas, on the other, the 'anaemics' believed in plenty of pillows under the head to drain the blood away.

An adroit inventor exploited both theories by devising a rocking bed—rocking end to end, not side to side. Better still, why not go for natural rocking—sleep on a boat—and there is all that ozone to which the Victorians attributed many therapeutic properties. Top-heavy wooden-hulled boats were ideal for bobbing about on the waves, and there were plenty to spare at the time because it was the era of the new iron ship. Easily converted into inshore floating hotels, these old boats had a new lease of life, attracting poor sleepers in their droves from far and wide, especially from the cities. Under the guise of when on a boat live like a seafarer, guests would be given a much appreciated tot of grog (rum) at bedtime—often in large quantities to suppress sea sickness because green and sickly guests carried down the gang-plank on a stretcher were not good for trade. A few nights of what usually turned out to be a ghastly experience and the person with insomnia was most grateful to part with their money and return home to sleep in their now appealing beds.

One of the most notable Victorians with self-confessed insomnia was Charles Dickens, who would take long walks at night when he could not sleep. Moreover, his recipe was to sleep exactly in the middle of the bed, with the bed head pointing to the North Pole. This is why he always carried a compass, especially as he believed that he also had to be facing north before he could write, because this would foster his creativity. Dickens was also a firm believer in mesmerism (we now know it as 'hypnosis'), which, then, was also called 'animal magnetism' and thought to be linked to real magnetism. This connection with magnetism probably came from the activities of Mesmer himself, who used pieces of magnetic iron ore, or 'lodestone', as part of his mesmeric treatments, including curing insomnia. Lodestones embedded in pillows became a very popular cure-all among the Victorians and, for reasons I cannot determine, lodestones were also believed to remove wrinkles. Dickens dismissed such use of magnets as 'unnatural'.

We may laugh at those credulous Victorians, presuming that it could not happen nowadays, but magnetic pillows and mattresses are advertised even today, and a 'magnetic field deficiency syndrome', with symptoms including insomnia, was a very popular diagnosis in Japan in the 1950s and 1960s. Alas, human nature being what it is, life does not really change, and the same gullibility as in Victorian times is found, one way or another, generation after generation. Daft notions about how to get a better night's sleep still abound. Although it is all too easy to be light-hearted about insomnia, the desperate attempts of today's insomniac to thwart that dread of bedtime makes them turn to all sorts of aids to sleep, many of which are unproven and costly. In the UK we spend over £20 million a year on 'over-the-counter' (non-prescribed) medicines to treat insomnia—some are quite good at helping sleep, but others are a waste of money.

Seniors

Whereas early morning awakening can be a key sign of depression, this is not so unless other clear signs of depression can be established, especially in elderly people. Moreover, this common sleep problem in older people is not so much a disorder of sleep as just another natural sign of ageing, if they are otherwise healthy. As creaking bones, white hair, and wrinkled skin are obvious signs of getting old, patterns of sleep and wakefulness also change with age. Many older people do not appreciate this and believe that their sleep problem is an illness, which it usually is not. Whereas younger people can remain awake for sixteen or more hours and then sleep for seven or so hours, this clear pattern becomes less obvious in older people, who often have difficulty in remaining alert continuously throughout those sixteen hours and have to take naps, not just in the early afternoon, but at other times in the day. As many senior citizens cannot sustain long periods of wakefulness, by mid-evening they are often very sleepy and retire to bed. Sleep comes rapidly, probably for around five or six hours, until about 4am, and they cannot sleep any more. That is it, unfortunately: the full sleep quota has been taken, which is why they are alert and cannot get back to sleep, with brain and body ready for the waking day.

For healthy people, the daily need for sleep does not differ much between the ages of 40 and 80 years (take a look at Figure 14 in Chapter 14)—maybe only half an hour less in elderly people. Their daytime naps can easily add up to an hour or so, leaving only five or six hours of sleep for the night. With the early bedtime, all this leads to the early morning awakening.

To add to the misery, it is often cold and lonely then, because most people are asleep. There is little of interest on the radio or TV at this time, and so it is, 'I'll stay in bed and try to go back to sleep'. As time drags on it becomes, 'I still can't sleep—there must be something wrong with me'. Eventually, after several days or even weeks, this all becomes too much and the person is off to the doctor, to whom they can give a very agitated account. The doctor may well mistake this distress, together with the early morning awakening, as a sign of depression, prescribe an antidepressant drug, and maybe sleeping pills. Not surprisingly, the antidepressants do not work too well, because the patient is not really depressed. Moreover, the sleeping pills may create more problems. When should the tablet be taken—at the beginning of the night when it is not needed, because going to sleep is not the difficulty? In which case, a relatively higher dose is required so that the effect is sustained beyond the five or so hours when they would typically wake up. Or, perhaps take it after waking up early in the morning? Again, a relatively higher dose is required because more 'knock-out' is needed, as they are alert and their real sleep need is satisfied. An added complication (if there was not enough already) is that the ability of the liver and kidneys to dispose of these medicines declines with age, and it can be difficult to get the dosage right, and easy to take too high a dose. It is hardly surprising that all this can easily lead to daytime grogginess caused by carry-over effects of the tablets, an increased likelihood of falls, and more daytime napping—only to sleep less at night, awake even earlier in the morning, and decide to increase the dose! This vicious cycle can lead to even worse problems—in simulating senility and causing incontinence.

One practical solution to this early morning waking, and one certainly worth trying, is as follows. Instead of going to bed at 9pm, turn this propensity to nap to your advantage and do not go to bed then, but have another nap, in that warm and cosy chair, soon after having a cup of strong tea or even coffee. Keep the nap short, no longer than 20 minutes, and recruit someone or something for a wake-up call. Although the nap means 20 minutes less sleep, later in bed, it will offset sleepiness for around another 2 hours, even to midnight or beyond. The caffeine in that coffee or tea will help as well, kicking in after 20 minutes as the nap finishes. The delayed, but remaining, five or so hours of night-time sleep now provide a more acceptable waking time the next morning, when the rest of the world is stirring as well. And no sleeping pills are needed! Be warned—this new routine cannot be accomplished overnight, because the rather creaky body clock needs at least a week or so to adapt to this new, evening routine, especially as waking up after that extra nap can be difficult at first, but manageable if the nap is kept short.

Finally, for older people without sleep disorders, who feel that they do sleep too much in the afternoon and wake up early in the morning, plenty of daylight (even sitting by the window) or bright indoor light throughout the afternoon can be helpful, because this can both delay and strengthen the aged circadian rhythm. Give this time to work—a week or so of this 'treatment' is needed to reduce afternoon sleepiness, and possibly delay the onset of both evening sleepiness and bedtime, but, better still, it should shunt more sleep into the night—thus prolonging it. No guarantees, but it is worth a try and it is harmless.

'A ruffled mind makes a restless pillow'[1]

Insomnia—disorder of wakefulness?

We worry about our sleep, maybe unduly. In going to the doctor, even patients without a sleep problem will probably be asked 'and how are you sleeping?'—which may only be the doctor's stock phrase for breaking the ice, so to speak, but it reinforces the need for a 'good night's sleep' and 'beauty sleep'. It might even make the patient start thinking about their sleep and fret about it, or worsen anxieties over their sleep.

The National Institutes of Health[2] in the USA defines insomnia as:

> . . . complaints of disturbed sleep in the presence of adequate opportunity and circumstance for sleep. The disturbance may consist of one or more of three features: 1) difficulty in initiating sleep, 2) difficulty in maintaining sleep, or 3) waking up too early. (section 1, paragraph 1)

I am going to concentrate on those who have more chronic insomnia and have been suffering for at least a month. For about half of sufferers the reason for their insomnia is anxiety or worry, because there is no physical or more serious mental cause. It is called 'primary insomnia' and contrasts with the 'secondary insomnia' resulting from these other causes. Peace of mind at bedtime is the key ingredient of good sleep for us all, but, for one reason or another, many who have primary insomnia take their troubles to bed, are unable to unwind, and continually think about work, family, finance, or other pressures. All the hustle and bustle of wakefulness leaves the only time available for thinking about life, the world, and everything else to be when lying there in bed trying to go to sleep, when little else can be done to suppress these thoughts. All those worries that one was too busy to have during the day then seem to burst out and the mind starts buzzing. Trying to block them out by concentrating on something more pleasant instead, listening to music, or reading a book, can help or it can just postpone these thoughts until a little later and further prevent sleep. Worse still, the ticking clock seems to be getting louder and louder and the dial or digits on the clock face seem to become bigger and brighter—eventually the clock itself preys on the mind with increasing worries about not getting enough sleep.

This aroused, agitated state is not just confined to the night but can persist throughout the day, as one cannot unwind then either. In perhaps purposely 'keeping on the go' all day, this state of affairs pushes one's worries to the back of the mind, and is why I see this type of insomnia as a '24-hour disorder', not simply one of sleep, because it is really a problem of wakefulness rather than of sleep. One way to crack it is almost to ignore the insomnia and concentrate on sorting out waking life, especially as most sufferers obtain more sleep than they realise, because they are not particularly sleepy in the daytime, are 'bright eyed' by day, and do not complain of sleepiness—only that they cannot get to sleep. This type of insomnia, by itself, is not physically harmful to health,[3] although the underlying stress can have long-term consequences. Simply improving sleep by means of sleeping tablets is unlikely to deal with the stress,[2] and I return to this topic shortly. I should quickly add that those other people with insomnia who feel 'tired all the time' tend to have other reasons for their insomnia and I come back to this as well.

It is so difficult to convince the 'bright-eyed' insomniac that **no daytime sleepiness equals no real sleep loss**, despite what they think, and that they are probably getting more and better sleep than they realise. Maybe these people are sleepy after all, with underlying sleepiness being suppressed by being stressed and on the go all day? Or do they just keep busy, anyway? The evidence points to the latter. Apart from the anxiety, their problem also lies with a loss of the ability to realise that, during the first hour or so of seemingly endless tossing and turning, for what seems like interminable periods during the night, they are dipping in and out of what can be beneficial sleep. Sleeping tablets reduce the anxiety at bedtime (many are also tranquillisers) and 'coalesce' this fitful period into more sustained sleep, but it is not necessarily better sleep, because to my knowledge few sleeping tablets make people more alert in the morning—feeling 'better', yes, but not more alert. In a nutshell, 'more sleep' is not really the answer, here, but rather getting better wakefulness.

We are all prone to a modest 'dip' in the afternoon and this is not really a sign of inadequate sleep unless the dip becomes a distinct trough, with residual sleepiness pervading much of the day. A garrulous and lively person with insomnia is probably not someone suffering from lack of sleep. This is the first hurdle to overcome—trying to convince them that they will not become ill[2] or go mad through lack of sleep, because they also tend to worry unduly about other aspects of their health.

'Secondary insomnia' can be caused by pain (especially rheumatism and arthritis), other physical illnesses, and especially mild or more severe depression. Moreover, it can aggravate these other illnesses, and a vicious cycle easily develops. In this respect, 'secondary' is perhaps not the best description of this insomnia, and the more technical term 'co-morbid' is used, which points to this interaction between the other illnesses and the insomnia. The more despairing person with 'secondary' insomnia is more likely to be 'tired all the time', often miserable, and may feel rather worthless, and even angry with themselves and the rest of the world. This insomnia is more likely to take the form of waking up early in the morning, accompanied by misery and an inability to return to sleep, rather than having difficulty in falling asleep at bedtime. The worst cases are clinically quite depressed, look quite sad, and are certainly not bright eyed. Although sufferers may focus particularly on their insomnia, it is not the real cause of their troubles but just another symptom. Again, like the person with 'primary insomnia', simply treating the poor sleep, alone, is not the solution, because better sleep will come with tackling the 'co-morbid' pain, depression, etc.

If primary insomnia remains untreated, it may lead to depression and secondary insomnia. This is not to say that primary insomnia causes the more severe, secondary form, but, rather, that the underlying anxieties and other mental pressures behind the primary insomnia may eventually lead to more severe psychological problems, which in turn produce this more debilitating insomnia. Clearly, it is a case of 'a stitch in time saves nine'.

Anger and frustration

For the physician, primary insomnia can be perplexing, especially as the symptoms are largely unconnected with insufficient sleep, which is a key point highlighted by the authoritative report by the American Academy of Sleep Medicine,[4] which concluded (p 254):

> ... that no consistent picture of the daytime consequences of clinical insomnia has emerged. The ultimate significance of insomnia lies, at least in part, on such consequences. Current data seems to suggest that the daytime consequences which are associated with an insomnia complaint may not be due to sleep deprivation, but instead, to 'hyperarousal' [*over arousal*] which gives rise to both sleep disturbance and waking complaints. To the extent that this is true, it suggests that evaluation and treatment efforts might be most effectively aimed at this underlying arousal.

What is to be done? For a start, the sufferer must avoid getting angry about the insomnia and blame it for all their problems—it is probably the other way round. Successful treatment will come only when the sufferer focuses on dealing with the underlying causes such as the anxiety and worries, rather than on the insomnia itself—that is, when, 'oh for a good night's sleep' is no longer the centre of their life. A bad night's sleep is not the catastrophe that is often imagined, and you have to try to adopt a more matter-of-fact, 'here today gone tomorrow' approach to any apparent sleep loss. Besides, the sleep loss from those really awful nights is usually not as bad as it seems.

For certain, there is no point whatsoever in lying in bed in this state. Cannot sleep? Then forget it—abandon the bedroom, and go to another room and, if necessary, do the thinking and worrying there instead. If your problems cannot be resolved there and then, do something distracting. Distraction calms emotions and helps us think in a more detached manner. It needs to be pleasant and absorbing, preferably involving the eyes and hands, such as doing a jigsaw, painting, drawing, or making a model of something—even the Eiffel Tower out of matchsticks. Seems a ridiculous thing to do in the middle of the night when we ought to be sleeping, especially if one is not a jigsaw fan, and there are all those worries and problems to solve. Nevertheless, doing a jigsaw is more productive than just lying there worrying in bed, which is even more ridiculous and pointless. Watching TV, reading, and listening to the radio, even in the lounge and especially in bed, are not so good at distracting, because these activities are too passive, and the mind wanders back to those thoughts again. Hunting for those edges and pieces of sky in the jigsaw can be engrossing—making it difficult to worry. Besides, all that staring at those tiny bits makes the eyes feel heavy, when it is now an opportune moment quietly to go off to bed. By the way, avoid bright indoor lighting at this time of night—use a table lamp!

Many poor sleepers keep in their bedrooms all sorts of stand-by entertainments, which simply reinforce wakefulness—TV, videos, radio, books, and magazines. Some people with insomnia take a thermos flask of tea to bed—not for that morning cuppa, but as sustenance during the unwanted night-time vigil. If this is needed, go to the kitchen and have it there. All this paraphernalia of wakefulness only reinforces the association of the bedroom and bed with wakefulness, not sleep, and is why all of it should to be moved into the lounge, or wherever you do your wakefulness.

When, having done that jigsaw or whatever, sleepiness has returned (as it inevitably will), and it is back to bed, lie down straight away and turn off the bedside light. Still no sleep within what seems like ten minutes (the bedside clock has gone, by the way—I am coming to that)? Then, out of bed and back to the jigsaw. Do not worry about not having enough sleep—even if it is 5am and having to be up at 7am, you will sleep better tomorrow night. Above all, do not have a morning lie-in to compensate—always get up at the usual time, because this helps keep the body clock synchronised with both sleep and reality, as the odds are that this particular clock has lost its way.

Although various soothing techniques at bedtime can be helpful, such as relaxation tapes and discs of one sort or another, or more expensive 'biofeedback' methods for measuring muscle tension, the distractions just mentioned are equally effective, if not better, at taking your mind off matters. Furthermore, they are inexpensive and usually work more quickly. Many of these relaxation techniques incorporate breathing exercises, which can be helpful. One or perhaps two minutes of moderately deep and steady breathing produces interesting effects on the brain—the opposite to what you might expect.

Rather than provide it with more oxygen, the brain does not actually like this, because it upsets the brain's delicate workings. Instead, the brain reduces its blood supply to the extent that it over-compensates, and blood levels of carbon dioxide rise, causing feelings of light-headedness and relaxation, which can be quite pleasant. But you must not overdo the deep breathing—stop after two minutes because to continue further runs the risk of dizziness, fainting, or, unusually, even a fit. This harmless physiological trick is used at the start of many types of meditation and relaxation procedures.

Procrustes

A treatment for primary insomnia, popular in the USA, is sleep restriction therapy. The sufferer first decides upon their minimum daily sleep need, and when sleep should start—let us say seven hours and midnight respectively. This is a fair target to reach, but not yet, because, to begin with, two hours are subtracted, with an hour removed from either end of the sleep period—say, bedtime at 1am and arising at 6am. This is the only 'window for sleep' and it is tough at first—there are no exceptions; even if only three hours of sleep are achieved initially, it is still 'get up at six'. Perseverance is needed until undisturbed sleep fills most of this allocated period, and for at least two or three nights in succession. All being well, this initial regimen will probably last for only a few nights. The idea is that sleep deprivation builds up to increase sleep pressure, when sleep should eventually improve within this time window. Then, it can be widened by about 15 minutes, in stages, slowly but surely, alternating with earlier bedtimes and later rising times until the target of seven hours from midnight is reached. This rather radical treatment often works, but is not guaranteed, and is probably more effective if combined with other, more compassionate, treatments (see below). The most apt description of this method is 'procrustean', a word derived from both the Greek word for 'stretcher' and the legendary robber 'Procrustes' who fitted his victims exactly to a bed through either stretching them or shortening them by cutting off parts of limbs, as appropriate.

Tricks of time

The bedroom clock is the albatross of the person with insomnia, because clock watching only makes things worse. Do not worry about time ebbing away, and keep the bedside clock well out of sight, even though it is not out of mind. The only time one really needs to know is when to get up in the morning—set the alarm as necessary, put the clock under the bed, and no peeping.

How come most people with (primary) insomnia usually have more sleep than they realise—and why are they not particularly sleepy? For all of us, both good and bad sleepers, falling asleep is not like the bedside light—just simply switching off from wake to sleep. Instead, even a good sleeper begins by dipping in and out of sleep, with brief awakenings every minute or so, progressing with fewer awakenings into more sustained sleep. If these are short—for just a few seconds as they usually are, maybe just to turn over and get more comfortable, they are too short to be remembered. Everyone continues to have these brief awakenings throughout the night, around five times an hour, mostly to turn over. For the typical individual with insomnia, however, such awakenings at the start of sleep are usually longer than normal, to the extent that sufferers really do wake up, only to think that they have been awake since the previous, brief awakening. It is a trick of the mind; for them to know that they really have been asleep, sleep has to last for about ten minutes or so—much longer than for the normal sleeper who recognises sleep after only a couple of minutes of slumber. Often, there is worthwhile sleep, here, for the person with insomnia. It also explains why many of them are so certain about having taken an hour or more to go to sleep, when they may well have begun to have quite good sleep much sooner. Worries feed on these awakenings and, instead of the arousal being brief, as with the normal sleeper, anxious thoughts return to prolong these periods of wakefulness—seeming to make it eternal.

It can be so difficult to convince sufferers that, despite what they believe, sleep may well be sufficient and that is why they are not particularly sleepy during the day. They may become quite annoyed about this, sometimes unreasonably so—which is another clue, because there is often anger and frustration over other aspects of their lives, focused on when trying to sleep. Which is all the more reason for sorting out the personal problems and getting these other issues aired during the day rather than taking them to bed. Here is where good counselling can be so very effective, in highlighting these problems and demonstrating why insomnia is not so much a sleep disorder, but one that largely permeates all of wakefulness.

Keeping detailed sleep diaries, as people with insomnia often tend to do, logging for each night when and how they slept, is, in my opinion, to be discouraged. It simply focuses on the insomnia rather than on the real, underlying, waking problems. Besides, those bad nights of sleep, meticulously recorded in that diary, should be forgotten, not written down and kept as a constant reminder of times past. People can become quite irrational and superstitious about their sleep diaries, believing that if they do not make a complete entry for each night, sleep will get worse, and so further adding to their worries. Why not dispose of that diary by ceremoniously dropping it in the bin—better still burn it and that is that. Otherwise, one might lie there the next night, agonising whether to retrieve it, to aggravate the insomnia further!

Pills

Sleeping potions have been with us for thousands of years. One of the oldest acknowledged remedies comes from the herb valerian, named after the Roman emperor *Publius Licinius Valerianus* (AD 253–60) who apparently advocated its use widely. By the sixteenth century the more potent 'laudanum' was the most popular sleeping draught, and by the nineteenth century it was widely used throughout Europe and the USA. We know it today as morphine, but then it was also called 'wine of opium' or 'tincture of opium', comprising a mixture of alcohol, sugar, and opium. Famous 'opium eaters' such as DeQuincey, Byron, Shelley, Coleridge and Poe, as well as the English politician William Wilberforce, were really using laudanum, and not just to sleep! It was the main drug of abuse of the Victorians, and a good 'fix' was cheaper than a shot of gin or wine.

Today, as well as yesterday, sleeping tablets are not the solution to any form of insomnia, although they can be effective as part of the initial treatment. Besides, and as I have already mentioned, such tablets are unlikely to improve daytime alertness, especially if the person with insomnia was already fairly alert in the day. If anything, this alertness can be worse as a result of a hangover effect from the tablet, although this is much less likely when using the newer tablets. After a few weeks of taking any nightly sleeping tablet, whatever it is, few individuals with insomnia will actually have their sleep increased by more than 20 minutes or the time taken to fall asleep reduced by more than 15 minutes. However, as many of these medicines have the benefit of reducing the underlying anxiety and worries, this more relaxed state appears to make time go faster when lying there after lights out. Consequently, even if the sleeping pill has only a small effect in hastening sleep onset, it can make you think that this has happened to a greater extent and give greater contentment the next day.

Something like half the actions of any sleeping pill, be it a prescribed tablet or an over-the-counter herbal remedy, are the result of the 'placebo' effect and 'mind over matter'. Thinking that it will work can be a great comfort in itself, and help with relaxation. Belief in a treatment is one of the most powerful therapeutic tools. Many other 'aids to sleep' rely heavily on the placebo effect. Some contain nothing that actually makes us sleep, but are packaged and presented in such a way as to convince us that they will be very effective. There is really nothing wrong with this, especially if they seem to work, give satisfaction, and have no unwanted side effects.

Usually, a bad night's sleep leads to better sleep the following night, at least for that night, anyway. The poor sleeper may worry unduly about having this second bad night and, to avoid it, they take some remedy or other, and attribute the better sleep wholly to the remedy rather than to the more natural rebound sleep.

Sleeping tablets are a quick and easy short-term crutch, but not in the long term, because, apart from anything else, higher doses are likely to be required eventually. Simply knocking oneself out at bedtime with a powerful pill does not solve anything. However, if used in combination with professional counselling, which helps sufferers to understand and deal with their waking worries beyond the insomnia, sleeping tablets can be a helpful bed partner. Nevertheless, after a few nights, the best tablet is the one that sits on the bedside table gathering dust. Knowing that it is there, 'just in case', is almost as good as actually swallowing it. Not much consolation for the drug companies, however.

Peace of mind at bedtime is the real 'royal road to the unconscious'. Good sleep does not necessarily come with a new mattress, hop pillows, lavender oil, milky drinks, or a feng shui bedroom. If you cannot sleep then what is the point of lying there admiring the décor or expensive duvet; none will promote sleep unless we really convince ourselves that they will work—it is cheaper to buy that jigsaw, anyway! A relaxing bedtime routine helps—have a bubble bath (more about this in a moment), talk to the cat, take the dog for a quiet stroll, load the dishwasher, do the ironing, or read the paper. All help with winding down before sleep. Aromatherapy is popular—pleasant smells re-kindle pleasant thoughts and associations. A good aromatherapist will get to know the client and spend time in compassionate conversation, and the aroma can act as a pleasant reminder of the encounter—it is not always the aroma that may do the trick, but its pleasing connections.

Keep cool

In Chapter 6, I mentioned that at bedtime, before sleep onset, the body needs to cool down a little and lose heat faster than normal. Surely, then, a bath at bedtime will have the opposite effect and only make matters worse, especially for the individual with insomnia? No—not only is it relaxing, but, better still, and surprisingly, a warm bath helps cool us down even more. Although the warm water increases body temperature at the time, afterwards the body overcompensates and cools itself down even more rapidly. This is only by a fraction of a degree, but enough to promote a quicker sleep onset. It is why, having left the bath, pale-skinned people look particularly red—almost like beetroots—as the body is rapidly throwing off heat by shunting lots of warm blood through the dilated blood capillaries of the skin. The water should not be too hot, by the way—just pleasantly warm. Indulge yourself further with a bubble bath—it is medicinal, because plenty of bubbles act as an efficient heat insulator, preventing heat loss from the water's surface and reducing the need for a hot water top-up!

Beds that are too warm, especially those with electric blankets set on 'high', may be very pleasant, but they can prevent this cooling down and interfere with sleep onset, especially in poor sleepers. Some people find that it is not so much a warm bed that is comforting, but having warm feet, which can be encouraged by bedsocks—once very common. These seem foolish, nowadays. Nevertheless, they are worth thinking about, and who will see them once you are in bed?

Bugs and hygiene

Talk to people 100 years ago about sleep hygiene and the first thing that would come to mind is how to keep the bed free of bedbugs. This common scourge of so many beds is far from extinct, and is showing a resurgence. It is a ghastly, flat, oval-shaped, wingless, blood-sucking louse about six millimetres long that runs on a bed at an amazing speed. It can suck out its own weight in blood from your skin in five minutes, and then scuttle off to hide for up to six months, between meals. Infested beds would leave victims covered in irritating bites. Sleep hygiene, then, consisted of keeping beds away from the wall, bedclothes off the floor, and placing the bed-legs in small cans filled with oil, like small moats, to trap animals running up from the floor. Mice find them a delicacy and, coincidentally or otherwise, bedbugs became more prevalent after the invention of the mousetrap and the introduction of the domestic cat into the home. Sprung mattresses provide a particularly warm haven for these unwanted bed partners.

Wishing someone to 'sleep tight' originates from the southern USA, from the days when, to avoid bedbugs, a bed usually consisted of a frame with a mesh of ropes strung across it, causing the bugs to fall through. To sleep well and avoid a sagging bed, the ropes had to be kept tight. In fact, 'sleep tight' is really only part of the saying, because one would wish the sleeper, 'goodnight, sleep tight, and don't let the bedbugs bite'.

Nowadays, 'sleep hygiene' has more pleasant connotations, albeit still a rather unfortunate term found in many popular articles on insomnia. It is reminiscent of a clinical, sanitised sleep devoid of any appeal, as though insomnia can somehow be disinfected away. Nevertheless, much of what it covers is good common sense. For example, avoid coffee or other caffeinated drinks in the evening, or even earlier. Caffeine can give some people too much of a 'buzz', as will heavy exercise late evening. Also to be avoided is alcohol, which is no friend of the person with insomnia, except maybe in moderation, as a small 'nightcap'. By small I mean only one unit, whether it be a single measure of spirit, a small beer, an even smaller glass of wine, or a little glass of sherry—drunk slowly when sitting and relaxing, before bedtime, just like that milky drink—or maybe pop that shot of whisky into the milky drink as well! Larger amounts of alcohol do provide oblivion, at least for a while, but not without cost, because this causes heavy snoring and other breathing difficulties, such as the obstructive sleep apnoea discussed in Chapter 21. What is more, as alcohol is fairly quickly disposed of by the body, if too much is drunk there soon follows 'alcohol withdrawal', a few hours into sleep, leading to agitation, anxiety, and waking up in a cold sweat—which, to be frank, is a mild form of the 'DTs' (delerium tremens).

Sleep hygiene also advocates avoiding daytime naps, because these further weaken sleepiness at bedtime. However, for those with insomnia who are not particularly sleepy in the daytime, they are unlikely to want to nap, anyway, and so this is rather pointless advice—more so for the younger person with insomnia. For the elderly person with insomnia, however, the afternoon doze may be inevitable and should be limited to less than 20 minutes.

Individuals with insomnia often have irregular sleeping habits that leave the body clock bewildered and not knowing when exactly to sleep. As this is such an important point, I am raising it again. For the individual with insomnia this clock depends on a constant get-up time in the morning, irrespective of whenever sleep finally began—even if it means a very short sleep that night. Unfortunately, extended morning sleep-ins are out!

Depression

One does not have to be severely depressed to suffer from the often debilitating problem of chronic, mild depression, which can go undiagnosed for many years. As I mentioned earlier, 'tired all the time' can be one symptom, but there can be physical causes for this tiredness, which is why people with it need to be checked out by their doctors. For those sufferers where it is largely of a psychological nature, it is often accompanied by a sense of hopelessness, especially towards the insomnia, and often aggressively so—which only makes the situation worse. Here, the insomnia can become even more the focus and blame for all one's ills. But the real culprit is usually this depression, which underlies the insomnia, not vice versa. Typically, awakenings begin after about two hours of sleep, culminating in an all-too-early final awakening at around 4–5am, and an inability to sleep thereafter. Again, sleeping tablets, alone, are no solution here, because it is the depression that must be treated first, when it is likely that the insomnia will resolve itself. There are effective drug treatments for depression, but these take some weeks to work, which is why other forms of therapy, to bridge the gap, may be required. CBT, short for 'cognitive–behavioural therapy', can be of help here—but more so for primary insomnia.

Therapy

So what is 'CBT'? It covers a collection of various psychological techniques that are useful in treating disorders largely having a psychological cause, especially anxiety, as in primary insomnia. Combined with an initial, short-term use of sleeping tablets, it represents the best way not only of treating insomnia but also of curing it. Thus, CBT means eventual and complete withdrawal from sleeping tablets or, maybe, just keeping that single tablet reassuringly by the bedside, gathering dust, as mentioned earlier. Rather than concentrate on the insomnia, as some therapists might advocate, CBT ought to focus on everyday waking life, because it is through the latter that real success lies. Techniques within CBT are mostly a refined form of common sense, but need to be administered by a skilled psychologist who knows exactly what refinements need to be done.

In utilising CBT, psychologists use their own terminology. For example, talking to the patient and helping them to deal with their waking anxieties, and allaying unfounded fears about what they think might happen to body and mind without sleep, is called 'cognitive restructuring'. Going to bed only when sleepy and abandoning the bed when one is not is called 'stimulus control', and 'sleep hygiene' is exactly as described earlier. Various methods for 'relaxation training' are included, such as progressive muscle relaxation and breathing exercises. 'Thought stopping' is another, whereby unwanted thoughts are blocked, for example, by continually repeating a word in the mind, or better still trying to focus the mind on a common object, such as a kite, and then trying to imagine all sorts of shapes and colours for it. This can be too much of a struggle to accomplish and, to be frank, may be a waste of time because it would be much easier and more fun to try my distraction 'jigsaw' therapy instead! Another technique sometimes used is 'paradoxical intention', which could be thought up only by psychologists, and involves instructing patients to stay awake when they get into bed—the theory being that it reduces the anxiety associated with trying to fall asleep, and thus one is supposed to relax more and fall asleep faster—enough said about that one, and good luck to you if it works! Finally, 'sleep restriction therapy', as already described, has also been added to the CBT repertoire.

Earlier, in Chapter 17, I began with a quote from an editorial in an 1894 issue of the *British Medical Journal*. The editorial[5] also went on briefly to review (p 719) various attested remedies for insomnia, and with great insight and seriousness pointed out that different remedies suit different people, to the extent that one apparently effective remedy can be the exact opposite of another. For example, hot baths versus cold baths, hot drinks versus cold drinks, long walks (in bare feet!) versus sitting while attempting 'steady but monotonous counting' or 'the more difficult feat of thinking about nothing'. The unwritten implication is that one's belief in the treatment is paramount. The article concluded with what must be the most extraordinary account of a cure, originally taken from the *Glasgow Herald*:

> Soap your head with the ordinary yellow soap; rub it into the roots of the hair until your head is just lather all over, tie it up in a napkin, go to bed, and wash it out in the morning. Do this for a fortnight. Take no tea after 6 pm. I did this, and have never been troubled with sleeplessness since. I have lost sleep on an occasion since, but one or two nights of the soap cure put it

right. I have conversed with medical men, but I have no explanation from any of them. All that I am careful about is that it cured me.

The editorial wisely ends with the comment that, 'we cannot help thinking that some of our sleepless readers would prefer the disease to the cure. But if any should like to try it, may we advise that they should first, at any rate, follow that part of the advice which relates to the tea, and leave the soap part as a last resource' (p 719).[5]

Beds

The role of the bed in procuring a good night's sleep is a matter for debate, especially when it comes to insomnia. The secret of good sleep for the individual with insomnia lies in a happier wakefulness and better peace of mind, not an expensive bed. We are spoilt for choice when it comes to choosing a bed. Testing it out in a showroom, in full public view, is far from ideal, especially if one is self-conscious and tense. When we sleep soundly the body relaxes to a greater extent than can be attained in the showroom, to the point that what might seem comfortable then may not be for the slumbering torso—let the buyer beware!

In earlier civilisations, and for most people, a bed was little more than straw on the floor with a pillow or neck support consisting of an animal skin rolled with the hair or fur on the inside. In seventeenth-century Europe and the USA, the typical bed was a simple timber frame with rope or leather supports, often with a bag of straw or wool used as a mattress. More comfortable frames would have a canvas or sailcloth mattress with eyelets along the edges, tied to pegs along the frame. In contrast, and for the more affluent, the bed used to be a most important piece of furniture and a status symbol, with beds and bedchambers also used as a place to eat meals and entertain socially. For example, 300 or so years ago, 'gentlemen' and 'ladies' had four-poster beds ('testors') on cabriole legs, with ornately carved upper supports and footposts. Their more luxurious mattresses were made from a mixture of horsehair, coconut fibre, and wool. The whole bed was surrounded by drapes or heavy curtains in the winter, to keep out the draughts and to ensure some privacy. These were replaced by lighter curtains for the summer. The hapless manservant or maid-servant, ever on call, would sleep in the same room as their respective master or mistress, but on a 'truckle bed'. It was a simple, low bed-frame on wheels, with only a straw mattress, which could be rolled under the main bed during the day to conceal its unsightly appearance. The less wealthy at that time would sleep on a simpler, less ornate four-poster, called a 'pencil bed', because of the plain looks and absence of carvings.

Tufted or buttoned mattresses, to hold the fillings and cover together, did not appear until the nineteenth century, and nor did the iron bedstead. The spiral steel coil bedspring first appeared in 1885, invented by the American, J.P. Leggett. It was unpopular at first, and by 1902 the inventor was on the verge of bankruptcy.

More contemporary mattresses made of latex rubber (Dunlopillow) or 'pocket springs' began to emerge in the 1930s. On the other hand, waterbeds date back to ancient times, to Persia, 3,600 years ago, and comprised several goat skins filled with water. The 'modern' water bed was evident as early as 1873, with the most notable being a design by Mr Neil Arnott, with its first recorded use at St Bartholomew's Hospital, London, as a treatment and prevention of bed sores. The idea soon became widespread, and by 1895 waterbeds looking like huge rubber hot-water bottles were being sold by mail order from Harrods, the London store. Unfortunately, the rubber perished and the inevitable bedroom disasters soon led to their disappearance until the 1960s, with the invention of vinyl.

The most famous and arguably the oldest and grandest existing bed is the 'Great Bed of Ware'. Not surprisingly it was made at Ware, England, in about 1590 during the reign of Elizabeth I. It is now located at London's Victoria and Albert Museum, and measures 11 feet (3.3 metres) by 10 feet (3 metres) and was built by a Hertfordshire carpenter, Jonas Fosbrooke. Mentioned in Shakespeare's *Twelfth Night* (Act iii, Scene 2), it spent much of its existence at the White Hart Inn at Ware, where it could sleep up to 12 willing guests at once—at the time, nothing amiss was seen in so many travellers and strangers sharing a bed.

Soft-sprung mattresses have become really popular only in the last 50 years, and most of us would be amazed by the apparent discomfort of the unsprung horsehair and cotton mattresses commonly used by so many people only a few generations ago. Nevertheless, most people not living in the western world still sleep on such 'minimal' mattresses, seemingly in total comfort. Our over-indulgence with soft mattresses is often claimed to 'underlie' what appears to be the increasing prevalence of back and joint pains. Although many sufferers have been told and literally sold the idea that a very firm ('orthopaedic') mattress helps alleviate these pains, there are no 'hard' scientific facts to support this notion. If anything, the evidence shows that a medium firm mattress is of greater benefit, cheaper to buy, and more comfortable, and leads to less pain in bed and easier getting out of it the next morning.

21 Snoring, gasping, and jumping

Breathtaking

John Wesley Hardin, the notorious gunfighter of the American Wild West, is said to have been so annoyed by the snoring of a fellow hotel guest that he went into the room and shot the hapless man dead. This is rather an extreme method of curing snoring, but the volume of some people's snoring can exceed 90 decibels (dB), louder than a road drill. No wonder that spouses are driven to sleep elsewhere.

Everyone snores to some extent. It centres on the upper airway at the back of the throat, called the 'oropharynx', which is a tube lined by various muscles, including those of the soft palate and tongue. Sleep causes these muscles to relax, so that the oropharynx sags inwards with the suction of breath when we breathe in. Normally, we sleep with the mouth shut, which clamps the tongue to the roof of the mouth, thus stopping the tongue slipping back and further obstructing the throat. Sleeping with the mouth open allows the tongue to move back to reduce the sagging airway further, causing these floppy bits to vibrate loudly with each inhalation, and the result is snoring. This type of snoring is usually harmless, and often troubles others more than the snorers, who are usually quite oblivious to the fact that they are the only individuals in the house able to sleep through the noise.

Yet snoring can be more than an annoyance. Sometimes the sagging of the oropharynx can develop into a total inward collapse of the airway, so that the sleeper becomes throttled and unable to breath—a condition called 'obstructive sleep apnoea' or OSA for short ('apnoea' comes from the Greek for 'without breath'). Needless to say, OSA can grossly disturb sleep and lead to excessive sleepiness, sleep-related accidents, and, quite possibly, a chronic form of hypertension (high blood pressure—see later). Thus, snoring can become a potential killer. During OSA, the sufferer is still asleep, and tries to regain breath with great heaving of the rib cage and diaphragm. These attempts only make matters worse—trying to breath against a gag causes abnormal changes to air pressure in the lungs, and impairs the flow of blood within the chest, heart, and lungs. Blood pressure soars during the episode and the heart starts to beat irregularly. Levels of oxygen in the blood fall, further affecting the heart, which needs plenty of oxygen in order to contract normally. People with advanced disease of the heart and circulatory system may die at this point. After about 15 seconds or even longer in this apnoeic state, centres in the brain that control breathing alert the rest of the brain to the emergency and the individual starts to wake up. This partial wakefulness restores the muscle tone in the oropharynx, which opens up with a massive inrush of air into the lungs to produce a loud choking gasp-cum-snore, heard as the ineptly named 'heroic snore'. Over the next 10 seconds or so, during milder snores or even normal breathing, the level of oxygen in the blood returns to normal and full sleep resumes. Although the whole cycle may last less than half a minute, it usually repeats itself many times. In very severe cases of OSA, several hundred such apnoeas and awakenings may occur during a single night—one or two a minute is not unusual.

These brief arousals are too short to be remembered and largely go unnoticed even in the worst sufferer, to the extent that this snorer often reports having slept well. It is why they are usually puzzled by their excessive sleepiness during the day, and are oblivious to the fact that their sleep has been so grossly disturbed. Not so long ago, the snoring would easily be overlooked by the unenlightened doctor, and the snorer would mistakenly be referred to a psychiatrist or neurologist in the belief that the excessive sleepiness had a psychological cause or might indicate brain disease. Nowadays, there are specialist sleep disorder clinics to assess and treat this problem, which is no laughing matter.

Snoring becomes more common with ageing, with about half of both men and women over the age of 65 years noticeably snoring at night, but this is usually harmless and only a minority experience actual OSA to any serious extent. In people over the age of 50 years, full-blown OSA affects more men than women. About half of these sufferers are obese, because the weight of the fat around the throat and torso adds to the collapse of the oropharynx, especially when the person sleeps on his or her back. Sleeping on the side can help somewhat, but does not prevent the condition. Often, a collar size of greater than 18 inches (46 cm) in a man of average height indicates obesity and potential problems with OSA. Having a large belly also promotes OSA, where it is not so much the fat under the waistline skin that is the problem, but the accompanying large masses of fat within the abdominal cavity that lead to these breathing difficulties.

For leaner individuals, other factors contributing to OSA include a small lower jaw that pushes the tongue backwards, enlarged tonsils, a deformed palate, and an excess of folds in the mucous membranes that lie on either side of the oropharynx. A blocked nose as a result of a cold, chronic catarrh, nasal polyps (growths), or a previously broken nose (rugby players and boxers are particularly prone to this) causes people to sleep with their mouth open, leading to the effects mentioned. Badly fitting dentures may worsen the condition because they can strain the oropharyngeal muscles in the daytime so that removal of dentures at bedtime causes an unusual relaxation of these muscles during the night.

Very heavy snoring accompanied by excessive daytime sleepiness usually points to OSA, but a proper diagnosis can be made confidently only in a clinic specialising in sleep disorders, after measurement of levels of oxygen in the blood during sleep, and often the breathing pattern as well. Unfortunately, although there are numerous sleep clinics in the USA, usually with several in every large city, there are still far too few in the UK. In the USA, doctors tend to view OSA as serious when the numbers of apnoeas per night exceed about 35 over 7 hours of sleep. However, the length of each apnoea is often of greater concern because, for example, 10 lengthy apnoeas may be more serious than 35 short ones.

Obstructive sleep apnoea can cause high blood pressure (hypertension) because the rise in blood pressure that occurs during each apnoeic episode can eventually extend into the waking hours as a permanent rise in blood pressure. This is more likely in those people having a form of hypertension that is resistant to drug treatment. Although obesity can be the culprit for both hypertension and OSA, only about half of those who have both complaints are overweight, because lean patients with OSA can still suffer from hypertension, especially those who smoke. The issue of whether OSA causes heart disease, apart from hypertension, is still controversial, but it must at least aggravate these disorders. About ten per cent of OSA sufferers have angina or arterial disease in the legs, compared with five per cent of similarly aged non-snorers, even when body weight and smoking are taken into account. However, I do not want to be alarmist over all this, because most sufferers with OSA have normal blood pressure and heart function for their age.

William Howard Taft, President of the USA from 1909 until 1913, is generally considered to be among the least successful of all American presidents. While in office, Taft was habitually falling asleep at his desk when reading papers and on many an official occasion when seated and meeting dignitaries. He would seldom go to the theatre because he would invariably fall asleep and miss the denouement. His private secretary would constantly nudge him and developed a persistent, loud but 'diplomatic' cough. Taft, almost 6 feet tall and weighing 335 pounds (24 stone or 152 kg), was quite rotund, to the extent that he frequently became stuck in his bathtub. More to the point, he was a noted loud snorer. Although it is disputed whether his hapless presidency was caused by this apparent OSA, shortly after leaving office he went on a strict diet, supervised by a Dr Yorke-Davies, an English physician, and lost 70 pounds (32 kg), when his excessive sleepiness disappeared. Soon afterwards he became Chief Justice of the US Supreme Court for a very successful nine years.

The point of this tale is that, if he did have severe OSA, as was likely, then whatever intellectual impairments he may have had as a result of this during his presidency, these seemed to have been reversed, as testified by his subsequent success. Nevertheless, contemporary research is now showing that OSA may impair the function of the brain, not simply because of the daytime sleepiness, but because of some brain damage. The countless episodes when the brain's supply of oxygen is reduced, night after night, must eventually take some sort of a toll. Comparisons have been made between the psychological functioning of sufferers with OSA with those without it, but with narcolepsy, which causes similar levels of excessive daytime sleepiness (see Chapter 15), although not impairing the brain's oxygen levels. OSA patients have worse attention and concentration, in addition to some impairment to the frontal cortex, similar to those described in Chapter 8. Even with prolonged and successful treatment for the OSA, this brain impairment may take many months to improve, and may never fully recover.

Better news

What can be done to treat OSA? Numerous inventors have patented commercial versions of old folk remedies, such as the 'snore ball'—something hard, fixed to the snorer's back to deter them from lying supine. Other gadgets include mouth gags, muzzles, chin straps, nasal tubes to facilitate breathing and inserted up the nostrils, as well as special pillows and collars. Some of these methods may help people who snore mildly, who do not have OSA, but are fairly useless for those more seriously affected, especially any device that clamps the mouth shut when the nose is already partly blocked.

For obese individuals, the more sensible treatment is to lose weight, which will usually reduce OSA. However, this is easier said than done, and may take many months of dieting and exercising before sufficient fat is lost. For those people with enlarged tonsils and swollen throat tissues, or a damaged nose, corrective surgery can help. There is no really effective drug for treating OSA. Even though drugs that increase the tone of these throat muscles have had limited success, they do have some side effects. The most promising treatment to date is called 'nasal continuous positive airway pressure' or 'nCPAP' for short. It is rather like a small vacuum cleaner working in reverse, providing air into the nose via a tube to a nose mask. Air is provided at a slightly higher than normal pressure, which puffs out the rear of the throat and allows normal nasal breathing. It simply allows you to breathe on your own, unimpeded, and is not like a hospital ventilator, which forces air into the lungs. Throughout sleep, the patient wears this fitted nose mask and, provided that no air leaks out around it, and that the nCPAP pump is adjusted correctly, the higher pressure of the air entering the nose will stop OSA instantly. The mouth remains closed (without assistance), to keep the tongue in place. This nCPAP is easily used at home, and is quite portable for those nights away, although the sight of someone wearing the mask is rather off-putting. Nevertheless, the method is harmless and usually extremely effective. The improvement in alertness the next day, even after the first night on nCPAP, is usually dramatic.

A newer, less obtrusive, and often very effective treatment is a type of denture plate, which pulls the lower jaw forward, thus opening up the back of the throat. They also allow the jaws to close, keeping the tongue in place, and in doing so permit normal breathing through the nose. Although some of these devices can be moulded to one's teeth by softening them in hot water beforehand, others have to be individually designed and fitted by a dentist, which can make the method more expensive than an nCPAP device.

Gasping

During OSA, attempts at breathing usually continue, with the chest heaving against the obstructed throat. However, there is another form of sleep apnoea not caused by throat collapse, but when breathing stops entirely, and the ribs and diaphragm cease movement. This is 'central sleep apnoea', when the breathing control centre in the brain just switches off. Again, when the blood oxygen levels fall to a dangerous level, the brain momentarily wakes the individual up, when there is a 'gasp' (not a snore) caused by the inrush of air. As in OSA, the awakenings are usually too short to remember. We do not know why this happens, although, it is more likely to occur during rapid eye movement (REM) sleep. Some people with OSA may also have central sleep apnoea (CSA for short), which can switch in after a few seconds of OSA. The nCPAP is of no use to CSA, unfortunately, but drug treatment can help.

Central sleep apnoea may apply particularly to babies, usually aged under six months, whose breathing control centres have yet to develop fully. Even small obstructions to breathing during sleep at this age (such as a cold or regurgitation of food) can trigger a central apnoea. Again, emergency responses within the brain will normally rouse the baby to breathe. Some scientists suspect, however, that sudden infant death syndrome (SIDS—known more popularly as 'cot death') might be partly linked to central sleep apnoea. By placing the baby to sleep on its back, the risk of cot death is reduced by half.

There is a more minor type of central sleep apnoea during sleep, when breathing continues unobstructed, but when we do not breath enough because this becomes too shallow or infrequent, or both. It is called 'hypoventilation' or 'hypopnoea'. Blood oxygen levels fall or there may be other changes to the blood and breathlessness sets in. Again, there is a momentary awakening—normal breathing resumes and sleep returns. If it becomes too frequent, the sleep disturbance will also lead to daytime sleepiness. Hypopnoeas sometimes accompany OSA. There are various possible causes of sleep hypopnoea, which usually need the attention of the sleep disorder clinic to sort out.

Alcohol

Depending upon how much is consumed, alcohol impairs breathing during sleep in three different ways:

1. It increases the relaxation in the throat muscles.
2. It causes the brain's breathing centre to be less responsive to low blood oxygen levels.
3. It slows up the emergency reaction to wake up.

All can occur at once in the course of a night, even after modest alcohol intake, to produce the three types of breathing problem just described (obstructive and central apnoea, as well as hypopnoea). After having alcohol, people who usually snore only harmlessly (that is, no OSA) will probably suffer clear OSA, and those who normally have no signs of snoring at all will now do so, especially during the first few hours of sleep until the alcohol wears off. What is more, the ensuing hangover can at least in part be blamed on the apnoeas. Although a small nightcap can be pleasant, relaxing, and harmless to sleep, increasing the dose to induce sleep will only worsen matters.

When it comes to alcohol and sleep, it is indeed a matter of, 'a little of what you fancy does you good'!

Legs

Finally, I would like to turn to another, different but equally serious sleep disorder that is liable to cause excessive daytime sleepiness. We have all experienced that occasional 'waking up with a jump', soon after going to sleep. Usually, it is a kicking of one or both lower legs, and the real cause is unknown. For some people it becomes frequent and distressing, happening most nights every 30 seconds or so, especially around the onset of sleep and well into it. Each of these particular kicks lasts longer than the 'normal jump', maybe a couple of seconds at a time, as the leg muscles continue to contract after the jump. Needless to say, it is very unpleasant for sufferers who not only cannot get to sleep because of the kicks, but when they do fall asleep, unbeknown to the sleeper, kicking continues to disturb sleep, and does not abate until sleep eventually becomes deeper. Even if they do wake up, the kicking can still continue for a while. Depending on the extent of the sleep disruption, there is sleepiness in the daytime, which is often excessive. The sleep of bed partners can also be impaired if they are the recipients of the kicks. This complaint is usually called 'hypnic jerks', and is one of two related disorders that come under the general heading, 'periodic limb movements in sleep' or PLMS for short.

The other disorder is 'restless legs syndrome', which can also appear in wakefulness, particularly in the evenings, when it is experienced as an unpleasant creeping–crawling sensation deep within the knees, thighs, or calves, brought on by sitting or lying. Some people liken it to a feeling of 'insects inside the legs'. Typically, it produces an irresistible urge to stretch and move the legs about, which, when in bed, further delays sleep onset. Similar to hypnic jerks, it continues into sleep, causing momentary awakenings and sleep disruption. Sufferers can obtain some relief by getting out of bed and walking about. Even keeping the legs and feet cool can give some relief.

Both hypnic jerks and restless legs are more common during pregnancy, in the over-50s, and more so in elderly people. Sufferers may well need the attention of a sleep clinic for proper diagnosis and treatment. One or both forms can appear with: iron deficiency, a build-up of urea in the blood, heavy smoking, or excessive caffeine intake, and as a side effect of a wide range of drugs including some antidepressants and antihistamines. Apart from sorting out these aggravating factors, treatment for both disorders is usually by leg exercises during the day, iron supplements if necessary, and, most recently, medicines called 'dopamine agonists' which increase the

Table 3 The Epworth Sleepiness Scale

How likely are you to doze off or fall asleep in the following situations, in contrast to just feeling sleepy?

For each of the situations listed below give yourself a score of 0 to 3, where:

0 = would never doze
1 = slight chance
2 = moderate chance
3 = high chance

Work out your total score by adding up the scores for situations 1–8.

If you have not been in one of these situations recently, think about how you might have been affected.

Score

1. Sitting and reading
2. Watching TV
3. Sitting inactive in a public place (e.g. cinema, theatre, meeting)
4. As a passenger in a car for an hour without a break
5. Lying down to rest in the afternoon
6. Sitting and talking to someone
7. Sitting quietly after lunch (when you've had no alcohol)
8. In a car while stopped in traffic

Total

brain's own levels of the neurotransmitter dopamine. Of course, pregnancy will limit their use, although the mother with PLMS can usually be reassured that it will probably disappear after the birth.

As a guide to how sleepy people with a serious sleep disorder might be, especially those with sleep apnoea, PLMS, or narcolepsy, a simple, short, self-assessment test has been invented, and is used extensively. This is the 'Epworth Sleepiness Scale', devised by Dr Murray Johns,[1] from Melbourne, Australia. Easy to complete, it relates to everyday situations (Table 3). The scores are just added up to give the total, with the maximum being 24. Scores above 12 are regarded to be clinically significant—that is, something is most probably wrong—probably with sleep. This questionnaire is different from the other scale shown in Chapter 7, which assesses sleepiness as it is felt now, rather than looking back in time, as is the case of the Epworth Scale.

22 Children

What is normal?

Wide natural variations are found in the amount of daily sleep taken by children of all ages.[1-3] Take any 25 healthy newborn babies; although the average daily sleep for the group will be about 16 hours, one of them will naturally sleep about 10 hours a day, and another 19 hours—that is, one will sleep about twice the length of another. Parents of these shorter sleepers may while away the extra hours needed to entertain their progeny believing that short sleep is a sign of a higher IQ. Alas, there is no evidence to support this notion. By about 6 months of age, daily sleep would have dropped to about 14 hours,[1] with about 11 of these at night and the rest as naps in the day. Most babies under 6 months will wake at least once per night, usually more for breast-fed babies. Ideally they should be able to return to sleep by themselves, but often they do not—and therein lies one of the biggest problems, with more about this, shortly. By around 15 months, the daytime naps will be down to about 2 hours—probably with one nap mid-morning and another mid-afternoon. Moreover, the approximately 11 hours of night sleep ought to be without interruption or at least there should be no more than one awakening that needs parental intervention. Daytime naps are part of the total daily sleep need and, so the more the infant sleeps in the day, the less he or she will sleep at night. Too much napping can add to difficulties in going to sleep at night and the secret is to try to get the right balance between the two.

Regular daytime naps tend to disappear by 5 years of age (especially the morning ones), when the average child will continue to sleep about 10 or 11 hours a night and remain at this level until about aged 7 to 8 years, when sleep falls to about 9 hours. It will stay like this until adolescence when night-time sleep can easily rise to 10 hours, falling back to about 8 hours or so by the late teens.

I should add that all these estimates for sleep length are for when the child is actually asleep, and exclude both the settling down time from 'lights out' until sleep onset (which for 5–11 year olds changes little, and is anything from 0 to around 20 minutes), and the time lying awake in the morning, before getting up.

There is no 'ideal' amount of daily sleep for a child,[2,3] because there are these natural differences, as well as cultural differences. The key to children having sufficient sleep is whether they can get up easily in the morning, are alert and happy for most of the day, apart from a nap or two for the younger ones, and are not too grouchy. Children who are sleep deprived tend not to seem sleepy, but are irritable, 'overactive', seek constant stimulation, and are unable to concentrate on anything for very long. As we see, these symptoms are rather like a mild form of 'attention deficit hyperactivity disorder' (ADHD) and, before any diagnosis of this is contemplated, sleep should be checked out. Many older children do not get enough sleep, anyway, usually because they simply stay up too late, frequently thanks to the electronic entertainments in the bedroom.

Societies and cultures vary considerably in attitudes and practices concerning 'what is best' for children's sleep.[2] For example, in northern Europe and the USA there tend to be stricter bedtime routines and earlier bedtimes than in southern Europe and Latin America, where a more flexible approach is usually adopted, with children allowed to join the evening meals and family gatherings, only to fall asleep at some point, somewhere, and be put into bed. In these latter cultures the younger children will typically sleep in the parents' bedroom. There is no evidence to show that these more 'compassionate' practices are any worse than elsewhere in the world, despite what might seem to be a more erratic sleep pattern for the child. Of course, many parents with constraints on their time, who believe in strict bedtime routines and for their children to sleep in the 'comfort of their own bedrooms', will be aghast at these more liberal attitudes. On the other hand, the same dismay is expressed by these more liberal cultures about those 'uncaring' methods!

Off to sleep

With the USA and northern Europe in mind, and returning to babies, difficulty in their going to sleep is one of the most common sleep problems encountered by parents, causing much frustration and anguish. Whereas very young babies usually have to be almost asleep before being put successfully in the crib, by around six months of age they should be accustomed to being laid down awake. To continue waiting for baby to fall asleep in one's arms beforehand is inviting future trouble. Instead, after feeding and a quick cuddle, baby ought to be put back into the cot and allowed to 'self-soothe' to sleep. Cuddling babies until they fall asleep transfers the 'responsibility for going to sleep' from the baby to the parent, and soon they will learn that sleep is associated with mum or dad rather than themselves. Too many babies are unable to entertain themselves to sleep, either at bedtime or during night-time awakenings, and need someone to be present all the time until sleep onset.

Dr Yvonne Harrison, now at Liverpool John Moore's University, has made the fascinating finding that, by giving six- to twelve-week-old babies plenty of daylight in the early afternoon, through being outdoors or lying them near to a window, this improves their sleep at night and lessens it in the afternoon. This trick seems to help train their developing body clock and synchronise sleep.

For older infants and children, prevention is again better than cure, and the recipe for successful sleep, as well as for parental peace of mind at bedtime, is an almost unremitting pre-sleep routine set by the parent, broken only exceptionally and as a treat. It should be a period of progressive settling down, with the bedroom seen by all concerned as a place for peace and sleep rather than for fun and excitement. After the child has had a story and is tucked up for sleep, parents should leave the bedroom and not be open to persuasion to stay by delaying tactics ('just one more story')—kids can be very cunning at this and can have the parent well trained. The parent may even be conditioned into enacting various time-consuming bedtime rituals that, in effect, keep the child awake. By the way, babies and children should be accustomed to reasonable levels of household noises at bedtime and when they go to sleep—it is unwise for the house to enter into too 'hushed' a state.

Sleeping tablets/elixirs are seldom needed here, and at best should not be given for more than a day or two. Behavioural approaches in getting obdurate children back to sleep are generally more successful in solving most children's sleep problems, although parents must first reassure themselves that their child's awakening is not the result of genuine causes such as colic, milk intolerance (below), or real fears of sleep or nightmares, which require different approaches. Probably the most effective behavioural method in dealing with the young child who will not go to sleep at night is 'systematic ignoring'—although, of course, part of the problem may be that the child is simply being put to bed too early, so this must be considered. Nevertheless, provided that the child has plenty of tender loving care during wakefulness, and knows this, then this method is much to be recommended. After tucking the child up at bedtime, and maybe having warned the neighbours, the parent leaves the bedroom and resolves not to go back until the child is asleep, come what may. If the constantly waking child again wakes up, the parents should still ignore this or, at best, briefly enter the bedroom to reassure themselves that there is nothing really wrong, and leave immediately. If the child persistently gets out of bed and comes into the parents' bedroom, for example, nothing should be said to the child, especially when picking him up and putting him straight back to bed—repeatedly if necessary. Be warned—the first one or two nights are traumatic for everyone, and maybe the next night, but thereafter success is usually obvious and progressive. The distress and poor sleep for the parents during those first few nights can be tempered by their realistic anticipation of a fairly rapid and dramatic improvement in the sleep of all concerned. Half-way measures, such as the parents allowing the child to cry for 20 minutes and then intervening, are counterproductive because the child just learns to cry for this time, anticipating the parent's arrival.

Clearly, the success of this approach depends on whether the parents are prepared to let the child endure a few nights of what appears to be traumatic crying. If not, then there is, for example, the protracted withdrawal technique whereby, over what can turn out to be many nights, the parent gradually withdraws from the scene, for longer and longer periods, until the child eventually decides that remaining awake or waking up like this is unproductive. For the child who regularly wakes up in the night and is particularly demanding that someone accompanies him or her back to sleep, there is the method of 'scheduled awakenings',[4] which relies on the tendency for most of these children to wake at constant times. Here, the parent gently arouses the child about 30 minutes before they normally wake up, and then encourages them back to sleep. A return to sleep should be easy, because this is not on the child's 'waking schedule', and the usual awakening should disappear after a few nights of this, leaving the remaining awakenings under the control of the parent rather than of the child. The final step is gradually to stop these scheduled awakenings until the child no longer wakes and cries at night. This can be a tedious process, but is less traumatic than the quicker 'systematic ignoring' method just described.

Last, but not least, and assuming that the child understands what is going on, whatever method is used for ignoring the awakenings, there should be a morning reward for an uninterrupted sleep, to reinforce this 'good behaviour'. Largish, attractive stickers can be very effective, here, with the child encouraged to collect a set—maybe resulting in a bigger treat.

Night feeding

This controversial area is full of contrasting opinions and traditional views, where it can be difficult to see what is best. It largely depends on whether the baby is breast- or bottle-fed, because breast-fed babies tend to sleep through the night at a later age than those who are bottle-fed, especially if they suckle mainly for comfort, many times a day. Nevertheless, by around nine months most babies should be able to obtain all their food during the daytime only. A baby aged over six months, waking several times a night and requiring substantive feeds, is probably 'unusual', whereas one who wakes up once or twice for a short suck would not be. Large bottle feeds at night usually create or worsen the problem, leading to wet nappies (diapers), discomfort, and awakenings, as well as less feeding during the day. This type of night-time feed should be minimised or stopped. Probably the best way for doing so is gradually over, say two weeks, by decreasing the milk available (or breast-feeding time) at night, and increasing the acceptable time between night feeds. Success is usually marked, and parents are often surprised by how quickly the infant adapts. I am not a supporter of 'scheduled' feeding at night, by waking up the baby to feed them at a fixed time, because one cannot really tell when such feeds are no longer necessary.

Most children aged under five, who are referred to sleep clinics for persistent wakefulness and crying at night, simply have poor sleep habits, largely and unwittingly caused by the parents. However, a minority do have other causes such as nightmares and problems with digestion, including intolerance to cows' milk. For the latter, removal of all cows' milk products for a few weeks usually leads to much improved sleep.

Snoring

Some children snore heavily, to the extent that they have obstructive sleep apnoea, severely disturbed sleep, and excessive daytime sleepiness. This problem has been known since the nineteenth century, but seems to have been forgotten until recently. In 1889, in an article in the renowned *British Medical Journal* (29 September) entitled, 'On some causes of backwardness and stupidity in children',[5] Dr William Hill stated that the 'stupid looking lazy child who frequently suffers from headache at school, breathes through his mouth instead of his nose, snores and is restless at night, and wakes up with a dry mouth in the morning, is well worthy of the solicitous attention of the school medical officer' (p 711). Perhaps the most famous example of the time was Charles Dickens' 'Fat Boy', a pear-shaped lad who, in *The Pickwick Papers*, lurked about in the background, then always fell asleep, and whose symptoms have more recently been called the 'pickwickian syndrome'.[6] Although a fictional character (besides, Dickens never told us his real name), he was reported also to snore heavily and had all the characteristics of an obese boy with obstructive sleep apnoea.

For today's children, and apart from obesity, the most common causes of heavy snoring are enlarged tonsils, chronic throat infections, nose congestion, and hay fever. Unlike the somewhat older and clearly somnolent Fat Boy, younger children with daytime sleepiness can show unexpected signs. Although they have difficulty in getting up in the morning, sleepiness can appear as moodiness, irritability, inattention, impulsiveness, and even hyperactivity—all of which can be disruptive to classmates and impair everyone's schooling. Earlier, I mentioned ADHD, which I must emphasise is a disorder with a variety of causes, mostly unrelated to sleep. However, some (about 20 per cent) children with milder, apparent symptoms of ADHD can have a sleep-related breathing disorder as the underlying reason. They are usually not obese, but are more likely to have enlarged tonsils, causing them to snuffle and snore excessively at night. Often, a tonsillectomy can be the most appropriate treatment. Finally, I should caution that, although many children with more severe ADHD are poor sleepers, their poor sleep is more likely to be a symptom of ADHD, not its cause.

Nightmares

For most children dreams are pleasant experiences of everyday events. Nightmares ('mare' is an old English term for 'demon') are infrequent, often very real, and soon forgotten. But for some children they are very disturbing, particularly if frequent or if the child dwells on them for several days. It can lead to repetitive acting out of the nightmare with toys, a dread of sleep, struggling to stay awake, etc. Sometimes, frequent nightmares can be a sign of unhappiness, and worsen further if parents fail to confront and deal with their child's worries. One way to deal with nastier nightmares that are particularly distressing for the child is for either or both parents to take the child to a comforting place, such as the parents' bedroom, and ask the child to recount the dream. If and when the child gets upset during the recollection, it is best not to reinforce this upset by giving the child too much comfort or cuddling at this point, but to calm them down as soon as possible, while being supportive, and try to get them to carry on with recounting the dream. This sounds a bit callous, but the secret of success is to detach the emotion of the nightmare from the imagery itself, and treat the emotion on a more 'matter-of-fact' basis. Ask the child to go through all or just the nasty parts again, if this is not too distressing. When they have settled down, take them back to bed and encourage them to talk about the nightmare as much as might be necessary. If the child wants to, continue talking through the distressing parts in a dispassionate way, but do not dwell on the emotions—just the images. Each time the child goes over the nightmare, it will be easier. Do this again the next bedtime if necessary, especially if the nightmare is a recurrent one. Eventually, the fear of the dream should evaporate and the child is able to recount it in even a light-hearted way. This is now the time for parents to explore any other underlying worries and concerns that the child might have.

Whether one should place much reliance on trying to analyse the content of the dream in these respects is a matter for debate, but I very much doubt it. Usually it is no more than inspired guesswork, as in the case of adult dreams, with the time being better spent in delving into the child's conscious rather than unconscious mind. In more extreme cases, tranquillisers should be no more than a temporary stopgap at best.

Dreaming, as in rapid eye movement (REM) sleep, is naturally associated with the muscle paralysis mentioned in Chapter 14. The continuation of the paralysis into wakefulness is more common in children, who may wake up suddenly out of a nightmare, and find that they cannot move or call out for help. It may take many seconds to lift, and all the child can do is to breathe, move the eyes, and possibly, moan. It is very alarming and adds to the child's distress, especially if the dream imagery continues into this wakefulness, as can happen. Younger children may have difficulty in explaining these events, which only adds to the parents' concern. Happily, such experiences usually stop as the child gets older. Very rarely, this type of paralysis can make its first appearance in adolescence or young adulthood, when it may also occur at sleep onset or on morning awakening. Although it could be a symptom of narcolepsy (see Chapter 15), it is more likely that it will occur on its own, as 'isolated sleep paralysis'.

Some nightmares are not always what they seem and may turn out to be sleep terrors (see below) or, if accompanied by the same peculiar body or limb movements, maybe lasting for around half a minute, some form of epilepsy could be present[7]—in the unlikely event that this may be so, the child should be referred to their doctor.

Sleepwalking and wandering

When children are woken out of light sleep they will often report having been 'thinking' about that day's events—not so vividly and unreal as in dreams, but more systematically and ponderously. In deep sleep this thinking is less realistic and, sometimes, more disturbing mental events happen, with the most notable being sleepwalking and sleep terrors. These are related, but are distinct from the nightmares of dreaming sleep, largely because nightmares are the culmination of a long dream that the awakened sleeper can usually remember, whereas there is little, if any, memory for either sleepwalking or sleep terrors. The latter also tend to have some hereditary basis, because they can run in families. Sleepwalking is common during adolescence, but peaks before this and then usually disappears by the late teens. It can be triggered by anxiety as well as by sleep deprivation and anything that disrupts sleep, such as a noisy environment, pain, or discomfort. In susceptible children the worry can be trivial—the loss of a favourite toy, or just a frustrating day. Only in serious cases, when sleepwalking occurs frequently, might there be more severe distress and underlying emotional conflict, requiring some intervention. One of the best approaches in dealing with this in children is simply to reassure the parents, because, the more worried they become, the more this will be sensed by the child, the more anxious the child becomes, and the more likely sleepwalking will happen.

Children are particularly difficult to arouse from very deep sleep, and even very loud noises equivalent to a jumbo jet flying over the room can produce no response. Given that a sleepwalking child is usually in such a deep sleep, they are not only difficult to wake up when sleepwalking, but there is not much point in doing so, because it can lead to frightened bewilderment. It is best simply to guide or carry the child back to bed, especially as most episodes happen during the first few hours of sleep, when deep sleep is most prolific, and parents are usually still up and about. These children's minds are unresponsive to the world about them, even to a parent shouting 'What are you doing? Go back to bed'. Unfortunately, the uninformed parent might view this as gross disobedience and become even angrier, especially if the child urinates on the floor, which is not unusual. Foolishly shouting at or grabbing the child in return, which can happen at this point, will almost certainly awaken him or her, and the resultant commotion may wrongly be seen as a tantrum, with the child sent back to bed in disgrace and without comfort—hardly surprising that this only leads to more distress and sleepwalking over the next night or so.

Sleepwalkers, be they children or adults, behave like automatons with only a limited repertoire of behaviour. They do not walk around with the hands out in front, as is commonly portrayed, and have no memory of their sleepwalking the next day. Sleepwalking events can last up to 30 minutes, but usually average 5–10 minutes. Typically, individuals will sit up quietly, get out of bed, and move about in a confused and clumsy manner. Although behaviour becomes more co-ordinated, they tend to stay in the bedroom, often preoccupied by searching for something in drawers, cupboards, or under the bed. They may utter phrases that are usually incomprehensible. It is almost impossible to attract their attention, but if left alone they normally go back to bed. Navigation is done mostly by memory of the layout of the room and house, because the eyes are unseeing and usually it is dark. If the sleepwalker is asked to repeat the episode the next day, when awake, but blindfolded, they will soon come to grief because knowledge of the layout of furniture, stairs, etc., is now poor, although somehow heightened during sleep. Difficulties and sometimes injuries occur when they imagine that they are somewhere else, when familiar walls, doors, staircases, and windows are, in the mind of the sleepwalker, not where they should be.

If the child seems otherwise happy, but the sleepwalking occurs frequently, then pre-emptive waking can be tried, once more through the method of 'scheduled awakenings' just described.[8] Initially, over a week or so, a record is kept of the exact time that the sleepwalking appears, which is usually fairly constant. Then, for the next few nights the child is gently woken about 15 minutes beforehand, for about 5 minutes, comforted, and allowed to return to sleep. The likelihood of sleepwalking happening that night is lessened and, with the pattern having been broken, is less likely to return on the following nights when the child should sleep without interruption. However, all that might happen is for the sleepwalking to re-schedule itself later in sleep.

In older children, around puberty and adolescence, more adventurous nocturnal activities may occur, such as dressing and going outdoors. In this state the individual is seemingly alert, organised, and even able to get on a bike and pedal off down the road in the small hours. Clearly they can see and somehow know where they are. But this is not 'true sleepwalking' as such, because the individual is awake and in a 'confused arousal' or 'waking amnesia', which is sometimes still called by the old term 'fugue state'. Somehow, it is set off by a faulty awakening from sleep that can last for an hour or so. Again, the individual has little or no recollection afterwards. After the episode they usually go back to sleep, often not in their own beds, and eventually wake up in a strange place—fully awake this time, but bewildered because they cannot figure out how they got there. These are usually infrequent, often 'one-off' events that are still not really understood, because sleep scientists or doctors are never around when they occur! However, it is generally thought that stress and anxiety underlie them.

Finally, on average, and every other day, most accident and emergency units in large hospitals will see a child who has fallen out of bed, or climbed out of a cot and fallen to the floor, with about a third of them breaking a bone and another third with head injuries, which can be serious. From the nature of some of these injuries, some may be linked to the beginning of a sleepwalking episode. Of course most are not and, for those children more prone to simply falling out of bed, a low bed with sharp or bulky furniture kept some distance away is a prudent countermeasure.

Sleep terrors

These are another aberration of deep sleep, related to sleepwalking, and quite distinct from the visually vivid, prolonged nightmare, and are not just bad dreams. A sleep terror is a sudden and horrifying sensation with fleeting mental images that shock the sleeper into immediate wakefulness. It is also more common in older children than in adults, for which the problem is more serious (it was a typical symptom of 'shell shock' in young soldiers during the First World War). Typically, the child sits abruptly up in bed, screams, and appears to be staring 'wide-eyed' at some imaginary object—maybe 'a monster'. In this state, and often for ten or so minutes, they are usually inconsolable and quite indifferent to the loving intentions of the parent. Distressingly, they may even run around the bedroom. When all this passes the child seems to wake up somewhat, but is confused and disoriented for several minutes, and may well stay like this until sleep returns (which it will). Again, the child has little or no recollection of this event next morning. A sleep terror can develop into a sleepwalking episode, especially in the adolescent, when the terrified individual may be sobbing and walking around the house quite unresponsively for many minutes—half an hour or more is not uncommon. Again, morning recollection is fragmentary at best. If the child is otherwise untroubled, sleep terrors are seldom a matter for serious concern.

Fits, rolling, and rocking

Compared with wakefulness, sleep, especially non-REM sleep, happens to make the brain more susceptible to having a fit. One or two fits do not mean that someone has epilepsy, because everyone's brain has the capacity to have a fit, minor or otherwise, and some people are simply more liable to be affected than others. The child's developing brain can make them more vulnerable to this, and often they will simply grow out of it. For most children their only fit is during a sudden fever, accompanied by a high brain temperature ('febrile convulsion') when they are asleep. The brain cannot tolerate a high temperature, and that is why it is a good idea to get the temperature down as soon as possible, by body cooling.

Most of the fits seen in sleep are not the classic 'grand mal' form of epilepsy, which begins with stiffening body and limbs (the 'tonic' phase), followed by convulsions of alternating stiffening and relaxation ('clonic' phase). These two phases may last a minute or so, when breathing can stop, causing the skin and lips to become bluish.

Usually, it looks far worse than it really is. Tongue biting can occur, leaving a bruised tongue the next morning and maybe some blood on the pillow. Bedwetting can occur. Afterwards, the body relaxes and breathing (very heavy at first) returns as does profound sleep. However, most fits, being less obvious, last less than a minute, show little rigidity or convulsions, and largely go unnoticed—maybe there is only some vigorous twitching, stereotyped movement of an arm or leg, body writhing, facial gestures, and having the appearance of weird dreaming or sleep terrors with some shouting, crying, or wimpering.[7] There is some confusion and incoherence afterwards, when it is best to let the individual simply sleep this off. More often than not these fits are first seen as some sort of 'recurrent nightmare', but the accompanying stereotypical body movements in sleep suggest otherwise. Medical attention should be sought, although perhaps not that night, because there is usually no urgency and the condition is generally not too serious.

Rather strange, alarming nocturnal behaviours found in some infants and children, which seem like fits but definitely are not, are head banging, head rolling, and body rocking. Head banging is the most common of this trio, and consists of a forward—backward banging of the head into the pillow or mattress, or sometimes into a more solid object such as a wall or side of the crib. Head rolling is a repetitive side-to-side head movement, whereas body rocking is usually on the hands and knees, with a backward—forward pushing of the head into the pillow. All usually occur at sleep onset and during light sleep as well as in drowsiness, and sometimes in wakefulness. Head banging on its own is not a sign of brain damage or retardation, as is commonly and wrongly presumed, but can be found in healthy, normal infants. All these events usually occur with a rhythm of about 45 per minute, appear nightly, and last around 15 minutes or less per bout (often with several bouts per night). They tend to start at around eight months of age, probably do not have a psychological basis, and usually simply disappear by around the age of four. Children seem to enjoy this stimulation, and most cases do not need treatment, although the parents need to be reassured. However, if any of these conditions persist well into childhood, anxiety or distress may also be a factor, and should be looked into.

Bedwetting

This is a common sleep-related problem of childhood.[3,7] Children are not born with bladder control, but have to learn it. Whether bedwetting is considered as a disorder depends on where one draws the line for the number of wet beds per month. In general, children should have full control over their bladders by the age of four. Bedwetting reaches what seems to be an abnormal degree in around one in six children aged five to six years. If one or both parents suffered from this when young, it is much more likely in their offspring—but what exactly is inherited or acquired remains a matter for debate. Although bedwetting is commonly thought to have an emotional basis, this is usually not the case, unless it disappears for, say, 6–12 months and then reappears when there is clear emotional upset. Often the emotion displayed by a bedwetter is a reasonable response to the bedwetting itself. Unusually, bedwetting can be a sign of urinary infection, diabetes, fits, and even sleep apnoea.

Bedwetting occurs in all forms of sleep, and is not, as is sometimes thought, found only in unusually deep sleep. Many of these children have somehow not learned to recognise the signals of a full bladder, which would otherwise arouse the sleeping child. Psychological factors can be important, such as inappropriate toilet training, excessive teasing about the problem by siblings, or parents who inadvertently reinforce bladder 'immaturity' by continuing to keep an older child in a nappy (diaper) at night. Treatments depend on the cause, for example bladder training exercises, conditioning by the 'pad-and-buzzer' technique to enable the sleeping child to recognise a full bladder, and star charts for dry nights. Drugs are seldom the answer, but could be an occasional help during the treatment period (which can last several weeks) to give the child reassurance if sleeping away from home, for example.

Sleep talking and tooth grinding

Sleep talking, a minor peculiarity of mental events during sleep, consists of a muttering of jumbled words or phrases, having no real content, and usually appears in light sleep. It has nothing to do with dreaming. Sleep talking does not occur in REM sleep because of the muscle paralysis at this time, which includes the face and mouth (see Chapter 14). Sleep talking is common in adults and even more so in children. In fact, almost all children will do this if they are talked to during light sleep, when there is some sort of confused reply that has little relevance to what was originally said. If two or more children share a bedroom, and one starts sleep talking, then the curtain may go up on the bizarre theatre of the mind, because often the other sleepers will join in. None of the participants will be listening to the ramblings of the other, because each will be in their own world.

Tooth grinding, otherwise called 'bruxism', occurs in light sleep and can be alarmingly noisy. In older children (and adults) it is usually caused by distress or anxiety, although it can be related to jaw or dental disorders. Tooth discomfort may be why it occasionally appears in babies soon after the milk teeth have erupted. As to why it can appear in otherwise happy babies, remains a mystery. Clearly, it can cause much tooth damage and misalignment, and might require a special form of dental plate to be worn at night.

The teens—too late, too little

Once upon a time a child's bedroom was a place of relaxation for both parent and child, where the latter could settle down, perhaps play with a few toys with mum or dad, get into bed, and quietly fall asleep during a bedtime tale. Alas, whiz-bang technologies have brought inexpensive video games, computers, and mobile phones to the bedroom—for the younger child as well as for the teenager. For many, the bedroom has been transformed into a place of fun and excitement. Whereas it was 'oh no, not boring old bedtime', it is now 'yippee—let's go'. The bedroom becomes a battleground not only with the latest horrific computer game, but between parent and child in the 'getting me into bed and going to sleep game'. The fallback position for the child is the secret text messaging to friends that can be done on the mobile phone under the bedclothes, when the lights are turned off—thanks to the illuminated phone facia. Needless to say, late nights easily accumulate, with difficulties in getting up for school and the more subtle symptoms of moodiness, irritability, and inattention the next day.

In older children these effects of sleep loss give way to the more usual symptoms of sleepiness—being grumpy and falling asleep in class. Nowadays, late nights are becoming endemic among teenagers (largely thanks to the internet), who seem to think that they can catch up on lost sleep over the weekends, but this is not so easy, because sleep loss and sleepiness are more difficult to cope with at this age—much greater than teenagers realise. Worse still, if they persist with these late nights, the body clock will slip into this new regimen, and the 'delayed sleep phase syndrome' can set in.

This is not so much a problem of infants and children, but for adolescents, when it usually starts after a period of progressively later bedtimes. Whereas most teenagers catch up by having a few early nights, a minority are unable to do this, and develop a chronic inability to fall asleep until around 4am or later. The body clock is out of synchrony with reality, and delayed so that the usual daily peak of alertness is no longer early evening, but early morning—that is, they are chronically jetlagged, which is the reason why forlorn attempts to sleep at midnight fail. When sleep eventually comes, it is usually normal but falls well short of any minimum if they have to be up within a few hours to go to school—hence the excessive daytime sleepiness. If allowed their normal length sleep, for example, up to lunch time, or beyond, then they feel refreshed on awakening. This state of affairs can go on for many months, and is usually unresponsive to sleeping tablets. Sometimes sufferers are viewed by their doctors as being anxious or even 'neurotic'.

Treating it is best through 'chronotherapy'. As mentioned in Chapter 11, it is far easier to move the body clock forwards than backwards—that is, by extending the day rather than by shortening it. The treatment goal is to arrive at an earlier sleep time the long way round, by lengthening the day, ideally to 26–27 hours. It is accomplished by going to bed about three hours later each day, for six or seven days. For example, if sleep onset is usually not until 4am, then the successive bedtimes would be 7am, 10am, 1pm, 4pm, 7pm, 9pm, and ceasing at, say, 11pm, with bedtime held at 11pm thereafter—and do not let bedtime slip further. Up to eight hours of sleep on each occasion is allowed during the treatment days. Sufferers usually have no difficulty in going to sleep at these later times during the treatment, because it is well beyond the bedtime of the previous night, and they are usually very sleepy by then. The method is usually very effective, although the main difficulties are finding somewhere quiet for daytime sleeping, having to take some days off from school or college, and, as I must repeat, not allowing sleep to slip back again, afterwards.

Postscript

Often, sleep problems in children are not the problems of the child but of the parents, who may have unwittingly created the problem in the first place, worry unduly about a relatively minor matter that is inflated out of all proportion, or have transmitted their anxiety to the child whose sleep then worsens. As well as the child, it is often the parents who need attention, with advice and reassurance. It is remarkable how the behavioural problems with children's sleep can be resolved so quickly, by the right approach, and frequently to the amazement of the parents who, over months of anguish, become desperate for a good night's sleep themselves. Parents all too easily forget that infants and children are usually very adaptable and forgiving of what may seem to be short but harsh treatments given with tender loving care.

I sleep, therefore I am

The horizons for sleep research are still remote and, unlike this book, the journey through sleep is far from over for science. So where next with sleep? Certainly in the coming years we are likely to learn much more about how the brain controls sleep—from genetics, on the one hand, and from refinements in brain imaging technology, on the other, which will allow us to watch the living brain with increasing precision, to the level of microscopic activities of individual cells. We may find that there is more than a mere handful of genes influencing sleep—hundreds, maybe even thousands. But it is like dismantling an engine, right down to the last nut and bolt, and looking at the vast array of bits and pieces. How to tell which are the really important bits? Leaving out just one small bolt on reassembly may cause the engine to fail—but was that the vital piece that made it work? Or should we take a broader view and watch the intact engine running, adjusting some of the controls to see what happens? Perhaps a combination of both approaches is necessary. Even when we have found all the genes and the tiniest structures of the brain and its chemicals that influence sleep, as well as learnt about the effects of sleep loss or what happens when we take extra sleep, whether we will then know what sleep is really for remains to be seen. But, as Robert Louis Stevenson remarked, 'to travel hopefully is a better thing than to arrive'.

Will sleep provide the answer to how memories are made and stored? Probably not, because memories are mostly created when we are awake. But maybe they are somehow 'polished up' or linked up to other memories during sleep, to give us that different perspective next morning. Perhaps this is what 'sleeping on it' is really about. And what of the future for sleep disorders? Sleep apnoea will stay with us, especially among those who remain obese, and the problem of insomnia, too, will not go away. But cures for narcolepsy–cataplexy are likely to be found using medicines and gene therapy.

My own suspicion is that we will find that sleep is the meeting place for body and mind, where the mind interacts with the more subtle aspects of body functioning and can help the body combat disease. The immune system, after all, has close links with the brain.

A deeper understanding of the nature of sleep, along these lines, should underlie our whole approach to healthy sleep regimes and the management of sleep disorders. Yet much effort is put into shallow and temporary measures. The 24-hour society desires more wakefulness, while others concern themselves about insufficient sleep, despite neither knowing what sleep is really for, and persist in seeking out new medicines both to suppress and to enhance it. Elimination of sleep and sleepiness by a yet-to-be-discovered wonder drug would probably turn us into automatons, creatures of meagre routine, acting as soul-less robots incapable of self-reflection, empathy, imagination, coping with change, or meaningful dialogue with our fellows. Sleep bestows recovery for these uniquely human parts of our brain that allow us to become our waking self. They make us not just alert, a state common to all animals that are awake, but provide our self-awareness, and allow the human mind to work to its full potential. In a very real sense, then, we can perhaps declare: *dormo ergo sum*.

Appendix

Are you a lark, an owl, or neither?

1. How's your appetite in the first half hour after you wake up in the morning?
   - (a) Very poor [1]
   - (b) Fairly poor [2]
   - (c) Fairly good [3]
   - (d) Very good [4]

2. For the first half hour after you wake up in the morning, how do you feel?
   - (a) Very sleepy [1]
   - (b) Fairly sleepy [2]
   - (c) Fairly alert [3]
   - (d) Very alert [4]

3. You have no commitments the next day; at what time would you go to bed compared with your usual bedtime?
   - (a) Seldom or never later [4]
   - (b) Less then one hour later [3]
   - (c) 1–2 hours later [2]
   - (d) More than 2 hours later [1]

4. You are going to get fit. A friend suggests joining their fitness class between 7 and 8am. How do you think you would perform?
   - (a) Would be on good form [4]
   - (b) Would be on reasonable form [3]
   - (c) Would find it difficult [2]
   - (d) Would find it very difficult [1]

5. At what time do you feel sleepy and in need to go to bed?
   - (a) 8–9pm [5]
   - (b) 9–10.15pm [4]
   - (c) 10.15pm–12.45am [3]
   - (d) 12.45–2am [2]
   - (e) 2–3am [1]

6. If you went to bed at 11pm, how sleepy would you be?
   - (a) Not at all sleepy [0]

    (b) A little sleepy [2]

    (c) Fairly sleepy [3]

    (d) Very sleepy [5]

7. One night you have to remain awake between 4 and 6am. You have no commitments the next day. Which suits you best?

    (a) Not to go to bed until 6am [1]

    (b) Nap before 4am and sleep after 6am [2]

    (c) Sleep before 4am and nap after 6am [3]

    (d) Sleep before 4am and remain awake after 6am [4]

8. Suppose that you can choose your own work hours, but have to work five hours in the day. When would you like to start work?

    (a) Midnight–5am [1]

    (b) 3–8am [5]

    (c) 8–10am [4]

    (d) 10am–2pm [3]

    (e) 2–4pm [2]

    (f) 4pm–midnight [1]

9. At what time of day do you feel your best?

    (a) Midnight–5am [1]

    (b) 5am–9am [5]

    (c) 9am–11am [4]

    (d) 11am–5pm [3]

    (e) 5pm–10pm [2]

    (f) 10pm–midnight [1]

10. Do you think of yourself as a morning or evening person?

    (a) Morning type [6]

    (b) More morning than evening [4]

    (c) More evening than morning [2]

    (d) Evening type [0]

Scoring

Add up the points you scored for each answer (they are in the square brackets).

Score 8–12: definitely an evening type

Score 13–20: moderately an evening type

Score 21–33: neither type

Score 34–41: moderately a morning type

Score 42–46: definitely a morning type

Endnotes

Chapter 1

1. Sauer, S., Herrmann, E., Kaiser, W. (2004) Sleep deprivation in honey bees. *Journal of Sleep Research* **13**: 145–52.
2. Cirelli, C., Bushey, D., Hill, S., *et al.* (2005) Reduced sleep in *Drosophila* Shaker mutants. *Nature* **434**: 1087–92.
3. Tobler, I., Stalder, J. (1988) Rest in the scorpion—a sleep-like state? *Journal of Comparative Physiology A* **163**: 227–35.
4. Rattenborg, N.C., Mandt, B.H., Obermeyer, W.H., *et al.* (2004) Migratory sleeplessness in the white-crowned sparrow (*Zonotrichia leucophrys gambelii*). *Public Library of Science—Biology* **2**: 212–41.
5. Mukhametov, L.M. (1984) Sleep in marine mammals. In: Borbely, A.A., Valatx, J.L. (eds), *Sleep Mechanisms*. Munich: Springer, p 227.
6. Lyamin, O., Oryaslova, J., Lance, V., *et al.* (2005) Continuous activity in cetaceans after birth. *Nature* **435**: 1177.
7. Siegel, J. (2005) Clues to the functions of mammalian sleep. *Nature* **437**: 1264–71.
8. Rechtschaffen, A., Bergmann, B.M., Eversen, C.A., *et al.* (2002) Sleep deprivation in the rat: X. Integration and discussion of the findings. *Sleep* **25**: 68–87.

Chapter 2

1. Naef, A. (1926) Uber die Urformen der Anthropomorphen und die Stammesgeschichte des Menschenschadals. *Naturwiss* **14**: 445–52.
2. de Beer, G. (1958) *Embryos and Ancestors*. Oxford: Oxford University Press.
3. Gais, S., Born, J. (2004) Declarative memory consolidation: mechanisms acting during human sleep. *Learning and Memory* **11**: 670–85.

Chapter 3

1. Aristotle (350 BCE) *On Sleep and Sleeplessness*, Part 3 (translated by J.I. Beare): http://home12.inet.tele.dk/fil/slepless.htm
2. Legendre, R., Piéron, H. (1913) Recherches sur le besoin de sommeil consécutive à une veille prolongée. *Zeitschrift für Allgemeine Physiologie* **14**: 235–62.
3. Krueger, J.M., Majde, J.A. (2003) Humoral links between sleep and the

immune system: research issues. *Annals of the New York Academy of Sciences* **992**: 9–20.

4. Bonnet, M., Balkin, T.J., Dinges, D.F., *et al.* (2005) The use of stimulants to modify performance during sleep loss: a review by the sleep deprivation and stimulant task force of the American Academy of Sleep Medicine. *Sleep* **28**: 1163–87.

Chapter 4

1. Patrick, G.T.W., Gilbert, J.A. (1896) Studies from the psychological laboratory of the University of Iowa. *The Psychological Review* **3**: 469–83.
2. Gulevich, G., Dement, W., Johnson, L. (1966) Psychiatric and EEG observations on a case of prolonged (264 hours) wakefulness. *Archives of General Psychiatry* **15**: 29–35.
3. Von Kries R., Tosche A.M., Wurmser H., et al. (2002) Reduced risk for overweight in 5 and 6-y-old children by duration of sleep – a cross sectional study. *International Journal of Obesity* **26**: 710–716.
4. Gangwisch J.E., Malaspina D., Boden-Albala B., et al. (2005). Inadequate sleep as a risk factor for obesity: analyses of the NHANES. *Sleep* **28**: 1289–1296.

Chapter 5

1. Gillin, J.C., Buchsbaum, M., Wu, J., *et al.* (2001) Sleep deprivation as a model experimental antidepressant treatment: findings from functional brain imaging. *Depression and Anxiety* **14**: 37–49.

Chapter 7

1. Åkerstedt, T., Gillberg, M. (1990) Subjective and objective sleepiness in the active individual. *International Journal of Neuroscience* **52**: 29–37.
2. Drummond, S.P., Brown, G.G., Salamat, J.S., *et al.* (2004) Increasing task difficulty facilitates the cerebral compensatory response to total sleep deprivation. *Sleep* **27**: 445–51.
3. Broadbent, D.E. (1955) Variations in performance arising from continuous work. In: *Conference on Individual Efficiency in Industry*. Cambridge: Medical Research Council, pp 1–5.
4. Claparède, E. (1905) Esquisse d'une théorie biologique du sommeil. *Archives of Psychology* **4**: 245–9.
5. Dinges, D.F., Kribbs, N.B. (1991) Performing while sleepy: effects of experimentally induced sleepiness. In: Monk, T.H. (ed.) *Sleep, Sleepiness and Performance*. Winchester: John Wiley, pp 97–128.
6. Russell, H. (1891) *Yawning*. The Delsarte Series. New York: I.U.S. Book Co.
7. Mayer, C. (1921) Physiologisches und Pathologisches ueber das Gaehnen. *Zeitschrift für Biologie* **73**: 101–14.

Chapter 8

1. Landrigan, C.P., Rothschild, J.M., Cronin, A., *et al.* (2004) Effect of reducing interns' work hours on serious medical errors in intensive care units. *New England Journal of Medicine* **351**: 1838–48.

2. Report (1986) *Report of the Presidential Commission on the Space Shuttle Challenger Accident*, Vol 2. Washington DC: US Government Printing Office, Appendix G, p 2.

3. Harrison, Y., Horne, J.A. (2000) The impact of sleep loss on decision making—a review. *Journal of Experimental Psychology—Applied* **6**: 236–49.

4. Morris, G.O., Williams, H.L., Lubin, A., *et al.* (1960) Misperception and disorientation during sleep. *Archives of General Psychiatry* **2**: 247–54.

5. Bliss, E.L., Clark, L.D., West, C.D. (1959) Studies of sleep deprivation: relationship to schizophrenia. *Archives of Neurology* **81**: 348–59.

6. Harrison, Y., Horne, J.A. (2000) Sleep loss and temporal memory. *Quarterly Journal of Experimental Psychology—Applied* **53**: 271–9.

7. Kraepelin, E. (1919) *Dementia Praecox and Paraphrenia*. Edinburgh: Livingstone.

Chapter 9

1. Horne, J.A., Reyner, L.A. (1995). Sleep related vehicle accidents. *British Medical Journal* **310**: 565–7.

2. Miles, W. (1929) Sleeping with the eyes open. *Scientific American* 489–92.

3. Parliamentary Office of Science and Technology (2005) 'The 24 Hour Society', Postnote No 250, page 4: www.parliament.uk/parliamentary_offices/post/pubs2005.cfm

4. Philip, P., Vervialle, F., Le Breton, P., *et al.* (2001) Fatigue, alcohol and serious road crashes in France—a factorial study of national data. *British Medical Journal* **322**: 829–30.

5. O'Keefe, R. (1996) Sleep disorders and the Law of Torts. *Journal of Law and Medicine* **3**: 283–95.

6. Bonnet, M., Balkin, T.J., Dinges, D.F., *et al.* (2005) The use of stimulants to modify performance during sleep loss: a review by the sleep deprivation and stimulant task force of the American Academy of Sleep Medicine. *Sleep* **28**: 1163–87.

Chapter 10

1. Borbély, A.A. (1982) A two process model of sleep regulation. *Human Neurobiology* **1**: 195–204.

2. Bierce, Ambrose (1911) *The Devil's Dictionary*—available only online: www.thedevilsdictionary.com

3. Arendt, J. (1995) *Melatonin and the Mammalian Pineal Gland*. London: Chapman & Hall.

Chapter 11

1. Folkard, P., Tucker, P. (2003) Shift work, safety and productivity. *Occupational Medicine* **53**: 95–101.
2. Ingre, M., Åkerstedt, T. (2004) Effect of accumulated night work during the working lifetime on subjective health and sleep in monozygotic twins. *Journal of Sleep Research* **13**: 45–8.
3. Åkerstedt, T., Fredlund, P., Gillberg, M., *et al.* (2002) A prospective study of fatal occupational accidents—relationship to sleeping difficulties and occupational factors. *Journal of Sleep Research* **11**: 69–71.

Chapter 12

1. Horne, J.A., Pankhurst, F.L., Reyner, L.A., *et al.* (1994) A field study of sleep disturbance: effects of aircraft noise and other factors on 5742 nights of actimetrically monitored sleep in a large subject sample. *Sleep* **17**: 146–59.
2. The Actiwatch—Cambridge Neurotechnology UK: www.camntech.com/h_aw_1.html

Chapter 13

1. Steriade, M. (2003) The corticothalamic system in sleep. *Frontiers in Bioscience* **1**: 878–99.
2. Anderson, C., Horne, J.A. (2003) Pre-frontal cortex: links between low frequency delta EEG in sleep and neuropsychological performance in healthy, older people. *Psychophysiology* **40**: 349–57.

Chapter 14

1. Ladd, G.T. (1892) Contribution to the psychology of visual dreams. *Mind* **1**: 299–304.
2. Jacobson, E. (1930) Electrical measurements of neuromuscular states during mental activities III. Visual imagination and recollection. *American Journal of Physiology* **95**: 694–702.
3. Roffwarg, H.P., Muzio, J.N., Dement, W.C. (1966) Ontogenetic development of the human sleep-dream cycle. *Science* **152**: 604–19.
4. Siegel, J.M. (2005) Clues to the functions of mammalian sleep. *Nature* **437**: 1264–71.

Chapter 15

1. Nycamp, K. (1998) The effect of REM sleep deprivation on the level of sleepiness/alertness. *Sleep* **21**: 609–14.
2. Horne, J.A. (2000) REM sleep—by default? *Neuroscience and Biobehavioural Reviews* **24**: 777–97.
3. Siegel, J.M. (2001) The REM sleep-memory consolidation hypothesis. *Science* **294**: 1058–63.

Chapter 16

1. Aristotle (384–322 BCE) *Parva Naturalia* [*On The Sole*] (translated by W.S. Hett). Cambridge, MA: Harvard University Press.
2. Stewart, K. (1975) *The Senoi Dream People*. Toronto: McClelland & Stewart.
3. Domhoff, G.W. (1985) *The Mystique of Dreams*. Berkeley, CA: University of California Press.
4. Freud, S. (1933) *New Introductory Lectures on Psychoanalysis*. New York: Norton.
5. Jung, C.G. (1933) *Modern Man in Search of a Soul*. New York: Harcourt, Brace & World.
6. Kleitman, N. (1963) *Sleep and Wakefulness*, 2nd edn. Chicago: Chicago University Press.
7. Chaucer (1340–1400) *The Nun's Priest's Tale*. Harvard Classics. Cambridge, MA: Harvard University Press, lines 271–4.
8. Leonardo da Vinci (1452–1519) www.brainyquote.com/quotes/quotes/l/leonardoda135986.html

Chapter 17

1. Reyner, L.A., Horne, J.A. (1995) Gender and age differences in sleep, determined by home recorded sleep logs and actimetry. *Sleep* **18**: 127–34.
2. Monk, T.H., Busee, D.J., Welsh, D.K., *et al.* (2001) A sleep diary and questionnaire study of naturally short sleepers. *Journal of Sleep Research* **10**: 173–9.
3. Dyer, F.L., Martin, T.C. (1929). *Edison—His Life and Inventions*. New York: Harper Brothers.
4. Harrison, Y., Horne, J.A. (1996) Long-term extension to sleep—are we chronically sleep deprived? *Psychophysiology* **33**: 22–30.
5. Dinges, D. (1992). Adult napping and its effects on ability to function. In: Stampi, C. (ed.), *Why We Nap*. Boston, MA: Birkhauser, pp 118–34.
6. Husband, R.W. (1935) The comparative value of continuous versus interrupted sleep. *Journal of Experimental Psychology* **18**: 792–6.

Chapter 18

1. Editorial (1894) Sleeplessness. *British Medical Journal* 29 September: 719.
2. Terman, L.M., Hocking, A. (1913) The sleep of schoolchildren: its distribution according to age and its relation to physical and mental efficiency. *Journal of Educational Psychology* **4**: 138–47.
3. Tune, G.S. (1969) The influence of age and temperament on the adult human sleep-wakefulness pattern. *British Journal of Psychology* **60**: 431–41.
4. McGhie, A., Russell, S.M. (1962) The subjective assessment of normal sleep patterns. *Journal of Mental Science* **108**: 642–54.

5. Reyner, L.A., Horne, J.A. (1995) Gender and age differences in sleep, determined by home recorded sleep logs and actimetry. *Sleep* **8**: 127–34.

6. Kripke, D.F., Garfinkel, L., Wingard, D.L., *et al.* (2002) Mortality associated with sleep duration and insomnia. *Archives of General Psychiatry* **9**: 131–6.

7. Tamakoshi, A., Ohno, Y. (2004) Self-reported sleep duration as a predictor of all-cause mortality: Results from the JACC study, Japan. *Sleep* **27**: 51–4.

8. Ayas, N.T., White, D.P., Al-Delaimy, M., *et al.* (2003) A prospective study of sleep duration and coronary heart disease in women. *Archives of Internal Medicine* **163**: 205–9.

9. Ayas, N.T., White, D.P., Manson, J.E., *et al.* (2003) A prospective study of self-reported sleep duration and incident diabetes in women. *Diabetes Care* **26**: 380–4.

10. Aserinsky, E. (1969) The maximal capacity for sleep: Rapid eye movement density as an index of sleep satiety. *Biological Psychiatry* **1**: 147–59.

11. Punjabi, N.M., Bandeen-Roche, K., Young, T., *et al.* (2003) Predictors of objective sleep tendency in the general population. Sleep **26**: 678–83.

12. Bliwise, D. (1996) Historical change in the report of daytime fatigue. *Sleep* **19**: 462–4.

13. Spiegel, K., Leproult, R., Van Cauter, E., *et al.* (1999) Impact of sleep debt on metabolic and endocrine function. The *Lancet* **354**: 1435–9.

14. Born, J., Hansen, K., Marshall, L., *et al.* (1999) Timing the end of nocturnal sleep. *Nature* **397**: 29.

15. Bonnet, M.H., Arand, D.L. (2001) Arousal components which differentiate the MWT from the MSLT. *Sleep* **24**: 441–7.

16. Mavjee, V., Horne, J.A. (1994) Boredom effects on sleepiness/alertness in the early afternoon vs early evening, and interactions with warm ambient temperature. *British Journal of Psychology* **85**: 317–34.

17. Harrison, Y., Horne, J.A. (1996) High sleepability without sleepiness. The ability to fall asleep rapidly without other signs of sleepiness. *Neurophysiology and Clinical Electroencephalography* **26**: 15–20.

18. Graebner, W. (1965) *My Dear Mr Churchill*. London: Michael Joseph, p 55.

19. Hublin, C., Kaprio, J., Partinen, M., *et al.* (2001) Insufficient sleep—A population-based study in adults. *Sleep* **24**: 392–400.

20. McNair, D.M., Lor, M., Droppleman, L.F., *et al.* (1967) *Manual of the Profile of Mood States*. San Diego, CA: Educational and Industrial Testing Service.

21. Hoddes, E., Zarcone, V., Smythe, H., *et al.* (1973) Quantification of sleepiness: a new approach. *Psychophysiology* **10**: 431–6.

22. Anderson C., Horne J.A. (2007) Do we really want more sleep? A population-based study evaluating the strength of desire for more sleep. *Sleep Medicine,* (in press).

Chapter 19

1. Horne, J.A., Pankhurst, F.L., Reyner, L.A., *et al.* (1994) A field study of sleep disturbance: effects of aircraft noise and other factors on 5742 nights of actimetrically monitored sleep in a large subject sample. *Sleep* **17**: 146–59.

Chapter 20

1. Brontë, Charlotte (1846) *The Professor*, Chapter 22: www.online-literature.com/brontec/the_professor/22
2. US National Institutes of Health (2005) NIH state-of-the-science conference statement on manifestations and management of chronic insomnia in adults. http://consensus.nih.gov/2005/2005InsomniaSOS026html.htm
3. Phillips, B., Mannino, D.M. (2005) Does insomnia kill? *Sleep* **28**: 965–71.
4. Sateia, M.J., Doghramji, K., Hauri, P.J., *et al.* (2000) Evaluation of chronic insomnia. An American Academy of Sleep Medicine review. *Sleep* **23**: 243–308.
5. Editorial (1894) Sleeplessness. *British Medical Journal* 29 September: 719.

Chapter 21

1. Johns, M.W. (1991) A new method for measuring daytime sleepiness: The Epworth Sleepiness Scale. *Sleep* **14**: 540–6.

Chapter 22

1. Iglowstein, I., Jenni, O.G., Molinari, L., *et al.* (2003) Sleep duration from infancy to adolescence: reference values and general trends. *Pediatrics* **111**: 302–7.
2. Jenni, O.G., O'Connor, B.B. (2005) Children's sleep: an interplay between culture and biology. *Pediatrics* **115**: 204–16.
3. Ferber, R., Kryger, M. (eds) (1995) *Principles and Practice of Sleep Medicine in the Child*. Philadelphia: Saunders.
4. Mindell, J.A. (1999) Empirically supported treatments in pediatric psychology: bed-time refusal and night wakings in young children. *Journal of Pediatric Psychology* **24**: 465–81.
5. Hill, W. (1889) On some cases of backwardness and stupidity in children. *British Medical Journal* 29 September: 711–12.
6. Dickens, Charles (1875) *Posthumous Papers of the Pickwick Club*. London: Caxton Publishing Co. (Originally published 1836.)
7. Stores, G. (2001) *A Clinical Guide to Sleep Disorders in Children and Adolescents*. Oxford: Oxford University Press.
8. Frank, N.C., Spirito, A., Stark, L., *et al.* (1997) The use of scheduled awakenings to eliminate childhood sleepwalking. *Journal of Pediatric Psychology* **22**: 345–53.

Index